Manual of

Therapy for

Skin Diseases

Timothy G. Berger, M.D.

Assistant Clinical Professor
Department of Dermatology
University of California, San Francisco
School of Medicine
Chief, Department of Dermatology
San Francisco General Hospital
San Francisco, California

Peter M. Elias, M.D.

Professor and Vice Chairman
Department of Dermatology
University of California, San Francisco
School of Medicine
Chief, Dermatology Service
Veterans Administration Medical Center
San Francisco, California

Bruce U. Wintroub, M.D.

Professor and Chairman
Department of Dermatology
University of California, San Francisco
School of Medicine
San Francisco, California

Churchill Livingstone
New York, Edinburgh, London, Melbourne

Library of Congress Cataloging-in-Publication Data

Berger, Timothy G.
    Manual of therapy for skin diseases / by Timothy G. Berger, Peter
M. Elias, Bruce U. Wintroub.
        p.   cm.
    Includes bibliographical references.
    ISBN 0-443-08477-7
    1. Skin—Diseases—Chemotherapy—Handbooks, manuals, etc.
    2. Skin—Diseases—Treatment—Handbooks, manuals, etc.   I. Elias,
Peter M.   II. Wintroub, Bruce U.   III. Title.
    [DNLM: 1. Skin Diseases—therapy.   WR 650 B496m]
    RL 120.C45B47   1990
    616.5'06—dc20
    DNLM/DLC
    for Library of Congress   89-71271
                                                                CIP

© **Churchill Livingstone Inc. 1990**

Distributed in the United Kingdom by Churchill Livingstone, Robert
Stevenson House, 1–3 Baxter's Place, Leith Walk, Edinburgh EH1 3AF, and
by associated companies, branches, and representatives throughout the
world.

Accurate indications, adverse reactions, and dosage schedules for drugs
are provided in this book, but it is possible that they may change. The
reader is urged to review the package information data of the
manufacturers of the medications mentioned.

The Publishers have made every effort to trace the copyright holders for
borrowed material. If they have inadvertently overlooked any, they will be
pleased to make the necessary arrangements at the first opportunity.

Acquisitions Editor: Beth Kaufman Barry
Copy Editor: Elizabeth Bowman
Production Designer: Patricia McFadden
Production Supervisor: Christina Hippeli

Printed in the United States of America

First Published in 1990

To my parents and my wife, Bette, who have through four decades kept me growing with constant love and support.

Timothy G. Berger, M.D.

I am grateful for the knowledge of my colleagues, so generously shared with me, and for the reservoir of patience, support, and common sense of my wife, Mary, from which I so frequently obtain sustenance.

Peter M. Elias, M.D.

To my wife, Marya, for patience and understanding.

Bruce U. Wintroub, M.D.

PREFACE

The *Manual of Therapy for Skin Diseases* is designed to be an easy-to-use "how-to" book for the physician, resident, physician assistant, nurse practitioner, or student who must treat a patient with a skin problem. Although some diagnostic tips are given, the book will not guide one to the correct dermatologic diagnosis. It is assumed that the correct diagnosis has been made; the book then answers three questions: How should I treat? What should I do if the treatment does or does not work? What commonly goes wrong or is overlooked in managing patients with this skin disorder?

To use the text most efficiently, find the appropriate chapter in the alphabetically organized contents or in the index. Most disease entities are discussed in short individual chapters in a standard format. Some chapters begin with a brief introductory paragraph that summarizes the major points of evaluation before therapy or treatment goals. Because each chapter is reasonably self-contained, there are unavoidable redundancies.

Each chapter has four basic parts: initial therapy, alternative (initial) therapy, subsequent therapy, and pitfalls. *Initial therapy* outlines the treatment of the patient when first seen and can be termed "first-line" or "standard" therapy. These treatments are not absolutes; they reflect the author's preferences. *Alternative therapy* outlines treatments that can also be called first-line but that are listed as alternatives by the author's preference or because they are for specific subsets of patients (e.g., alternative antibiotics in penicillin-allergic individuals). *Subsequent therapy* describes what to do after the initial phase of treatment. If the patient has responded favorably, maintenance therapy, change in therapy dosage, or preventive measures are outlined. Also discussed within this section are treatments that may be used if both the initial and alternative therapies fail. The *pitfalls* section outlines common diagnostic and therapeutic errors. We hope it will help the reader avoid certain common mistakes. Also discussed in this section are the most common side effects of the drugs suggested as therapy in that chapter.

Unless otherwise specified, drug dosages are listed for the standard-sized adult with normal hepatic and renal function. Readers should check for drug dosages, side effects, and other precautions, such as drug interactions, in the *Physician's Desk Reference* if they have any further questions about a specific patient. When using the book we recommend that you read the whole chapter, not just a portion, before beginning therapy. When treating complex patients, you should not use this text as your sole resource. We have attempted to be as current and complete as possible without including excessive unproven or marginally effective treatments.

The appendices outline the side effects of drugs used commonly (e.g., steroids), or almost exclusively (e.g., retinoids), by dermatologists. In addition, we have provided up-to-date tabulations of available topical antifungals and topical steroids. Since the cost of topical steroids varies significantly, prices also have been included.

For the sake of brevity and to keep the book focused on its goal, two deletions were made. First, virtually no references are given. If treatments are anecdotal or experimental, this is usually stated. The current availability of computer-assisted literature searches makes it possible to locate the original reference easily. Second, in general, drugs are not listed in the index. Thus, the text cannot be used to find which diseases respond to specific drugs.

We would like to emphasize that this book is not intended to simplify dermatologic therapy or to teach dermatopharmacology. Dermatologic therapy is both a science and an art. In the text we frequently recommend referral to dermatologists for aid in management or for guidance in the use of specific agents with which they have more expertise (e.g., retinoids). With the information in this text, nondermatologists will be able to work better with dermatologists in the management of skin disorders. This may be especially true when dermatologists are relatively unavailable, as in geographically remote areas. Our goal is to provide information that will be useful to health-care providers at all levels of training. This may mean that the more advanced therapeutist will find some sections too simple; conversely, the less skilled may find some sections beyond their therapeutic scope. Therefore, we urge you to use the sections that your medical skills allow and refer when you feel uncomfortable.

We feel that the text will be useful for dermatologists both in practice and in training. It outlines detailed logical steps for the management of common disorders. In addition, it gives up-to-date guidelines for conditions that one may see only rarely in one's practice. Dermatologic therapeutics is a rapidly changing field, and many of you undoubtedly will have additional effective management strategies or therapeutic "pearls" that we have not included; we invite you to share them with us.

Timothy G. Berger, M.D.
Peter M. Elias, M.D.
Bruce U. Wintroub, M.D.

CONTENTS

1

Acne Keloidalis Nuchae

Dermatitis Papillaris Capillitii

This form of follicular inflammation with excessive scarring represents a keloidal reaction to prior or ongoing folliculitis. It primarily affects the nape of the neck of black men. Therapy involves treating the active folliculitis, if present, and the hypertrophic hair fragment-induced scars. These patients may or may not form hypertrophic scars or keloids at other sites.

Initial Therapy

1. Benzoyl peroxide gel or wash applied q.d. to the affected area.
2. Intralesional triamcinolone acetonide 5–10 mg/cc to individual lesions at 2–4-week intervals.

Ancillary Therapy

1. Patients should avoid greasy hair products.
2. Neck hair should not be trimmed short.

Subsequent Therapy

1. If active folliculitis persists, prescribe an oral antibiotic (e.g., tetracycline or erythromycin 500 mg b.i.d.).
2. If papules do not regress, increase the strength of the intralesional steroid to 20 mg/cc initially and then to 40 mg/cc if necessary.
3. It may be necessary to continue topical benzoyl peroxide and/or tetracycline therapy indefinitely.

Surgical Therapy

Most persistent or extensive cases are best managed by surgical techniques.

1. Few small papules: Individual lesions may be shaved off or preferably punched out and sutured closed.

2. Large plaques: Larger lesions may be removed by surgical excision. Scalpel or laser surgery may be used. Healing may be by secondary intention or by primary closure. If the defect is closed primarily, tension should be minimal to prevent a spread scar and keloid formation. A tissue expander may provide adequate tissue for primary closure of large lesions.
3. If surgical removal is performed, intralesional injection of triamcinolone into the scar may be required postoperatively.

Pitfalls

1. Avoid surgical procedures in persons who form keloids at other sites.
2. Discontinuation of the topical benzoyl peroxide and/or oral antibiotics may lead to a reactivation of the folliculitis.

TB

2

Acne Vulgaris

The initial evaluation of acne includes determining the type, severity, and location of the acne, and whether it leads to scarring.

Type	Severity	Location	Scarring
Grade I: Comedonal	Mild: Fewer than 10 lesions	Face only	No
Grade II: Papular	Moderate: 10–25 lesions	Face and trunk	Yes
Grade III: Pustular	Severe: More than 25 lesions		
Grade IV: Nodulocystic			

Acne vulgaris comprises two major types: grade I to II acne, which is usually mild to moderate, facial, and nonscarring and grade III to IV acne, which is often moderate to severe, involves the trunk, and may scar. Mild grade I or II acne that leads to permanent scarring may need more aggressive treatment.

GRADE I TO II ACNE

Initial Therapy

1. Primarily comedonal acne is best managed with topical vitamin A acid (retinoic acid, or tretinoin). It is available in cream and gel forms. Begin treatment with applications of the new low strength cream (0.025%) or 0.05% cream or 0.01% gel q.o.d., q.h.s. The frequency may be increased to q.d. after a few weeks, and then to higher concentrations (0.1% cream or 0.025% gel) p.r.n. Prescribe creams for drier-skinned patients and gels for those with oily skin.
2. Benzoyl peroxide gels or lotions (2.5%–10%) used q.d. or b.i.d. have mild anticomedonal effect and are good initial treatment for mild acne.

Alternative Therapy

1. The combination of benzoyl peroxide in the morning and vitamin A acid at night may be used when either agent alone fails. Its potential to irritate is also additive.
2. Mild comedolytic effect can be achieved by use of products containing salicylic acid 2%.
3. Removal of comedones with a comedone extractor by the patient or care-provider accelerates clearing. Vitamin A acid softens lesions, enhancing their removal.

Subsequent Therapy

POSITIVE INITIAL RESULTS

Once the initial response is noted continue treatment for 3 months. After this period, the frequency and strength of medications may be decreased at monthly intervals to a maintenance dose. Stopping therapy will usually result in a flare in 3–6 weeks if the tendency for acne is still present.

NO INITIAL RESPONSE

1. Consider the combination of benzoyl peroxide q.a.m. and vitamin A acid q.h.s.
2. Add an oral or topical antibiotic (only for inflammatory cases).
3. Consider more intensive acne surgery.

Pitfalls

1. Treatment of acne prevents new lesions, and, therefore, must be applied to the whole potentially affected area, not just the lesions.
2. Do not abandon any treatment sooner than 1 month. BE PATIENT. Continue treatment after a beneficial response has been noted, slowly tapering off until the level of therapy is at the minimum required for maintenance.
3. Acne will often flare after 2–3 weeks of vitamin A acid use. Warn the patient about it. It will resolve within 6–8 weeks.
4. Vitamin A acid may induce photosensitivity, so prescribe its use q.h.s. and encourage the use of a noncomedogenic sunscreen.
5. Overzealous use of vitamin A acid and/or benzoyl peroxide products will lead to skin irritation. Prescribe a dosage schedule and strength that will not lead to excessive dryness or redness.
6. Facial comedones (especially of the forehead) are often related to oily products applied to the scalp. Their use must be curtailed for the acne to improve.

GRADE III TO IV ACNE

Initial treatment is divided into that for mild to moderate cases (usually nonscarring and facial) and that for moderate to severe cases (potentially scarring and often truncal). Alternative and subsequent therapies are identical.

Initial Therapy

MILD TO MODERATE CASES

1. A topical antibiotic (erythromycin 2% or clindamycin 1%) in lotion or gel form applied to the affected areas b.i.d., or
2. Benzoyl peroxide lotion or gel (2.5%–10%) applied q.i.d. or b.i.d., or
3. A low-dose oral antibiotic (tetracycline or erythromycin) 250–500 mg b.i.d.

MODERATE TO SEVERE CASES

1. An oral antibiotic (tetracycline or erythromycin 500 mg b.i.d.–q.i.d.), and
2. Benzoyl peroxide gel or lotion (2.5%–10%) applied to the affected area. Patients with trunk lesions may find a wash in bar or lotion form to be an easier way to use benzoyl peroxide.

3. Use of vitamin A acid cream (0.05% for the face, 0.1% for the trunk) or gel (0.01% for the face, 0.025% for the trunk) initially q.o.h.s. may be added to the above therapeutic regimen. Encourage nightly application as tolerated. For trunk lesions, the vitamin A acid solution is an easier form of application.

Alternative Therapy

ANTIBIOTICS

1. Minocycline 50–200 mg/day is more effective than tetracycline or erythromycin. Cost limits its firstline use.
2. Trimethoprim-sulfamethoxazole 1 double-strength tablet q.d. or b.i.d. may work when other antibiotics fail. Its high rate of allergic reactions (6%) limits its use.
3. Clindamycin 150–600 mg/day may also work when other antibiotics fail. Diarrhea (potentially life-threatening) limits its use.
4. Prior to isotretinoin (13-*cis*-retinoic acid, or Accutane), dapsone 100–200 mg/day was used in very severe cases of nodulocystic acne with fair results.

ANTI-INFLAMMATORY DRUGS

1. Nonsteroidal anti-inflammatory drugs improve the inflammatory component. They are useful adjuncts to antibiotics.
2. Corticosteroids
   a. Short courses (7–10 days) of systemic steroids (prednisone 20–40 mg/day) will abort flares at critical times (weddings, proms, interviews, etc.).
   b. Intralesional injection of small amounts of triamcinolone acetonide (1.0–2.5 mg/cc) will lead to rapid resolution of cysts. Local steroid atrophy may result, so counsel the patient appropriately. The atrophy usually resolves in 3–6 months.
3. Isotretinoin: Patients with severe inflammatory scarring or nodulocystic acne will respond to isotretinoin in doses of 0.5–2 mg/kg/day. Pregnancy or possible pregnancy is an *absolute contraindication.* Isotretinoin should be used in females of child bearing potential only when all other standard treatments have failed. Pseudotumor cerebri, elevated LFTs, and hypertriglyceridemia limit its use in some patients. Side effects analogous to vitamin A toxicity are almost universal and are of mild to moderate severity. These factors restrict the prescription of isotretinoin to those physicians having experience with this drug.

Subsequent Therapy

POSITIVE INITIAL RESPONSE

1. Continue the treatment regimen for 3 months.
2. Vitamin A acid cream or gel applied q.h.s. is useful even in the most severe cases. Due to its potential to irritate and tendency to flare the acne, it is often begun 4–6 weeks after other treatment.
3. Topical antibiotics, although not initially effective, may be gradually substituted for low-dose (less than 500 mg/day) oral antibiotics in some cases.
4. Premenstrual flare and flares during college examinations and other stressful situations are common. Treat with additional oral antibiotics for 1–2 weeks before and 1–2 weeks after the potentially flaring episode.

NO INITIAL RESPONSE

1. Increase the dose of antibiotic tetracycline or erythromycin (up to 500 mg q.i.d.), or
2. Switch to an alternative antibiotic (minocycline or trimethoprim-sulfamethoxazole).
3. Add vitamin A acid gel or cream q.h.s.
4. Evaluate female patients for a hyperandrogenic state.
5. Consider the use of isotretinoin.

Pitfalls

1. Many failures in acne treatment are related to inadequate patient education. The patient must be instructed on what causes acne, how the available treatments work, and exactly how the prescribed medications are to be used.
2. External factors that trigger the acne must be removed for therapy to be effective. The three major ones are acnegenic medications (steroids, OCPs, etc.), acnegenic cosmetics and creams, and friction (e.g., from rubbing the chin).
3. Even the most effective medications take 4–8 weeks to work and sometimes even longer. BE PATIENT.
4. If acne fails to respond, perhaps it is not acne. Consider chronic folliculitides of other causes, and other diagnoses.
5. Female patients with acne, especially if they also have evidence of hirsutism, may have a hyperandrogenic state. Endocrine evaluation and correction or suppression of the condition may lead to improvement of the acne when other approaches fail.

6. Ask female patients whether they are pregnant or plan to get pregnant. Certain acne medications (e.g., tetracycline and isotretinoin) are contraindicated in pregnancy (see Appendix 6).
7. Ask female patients whether they are taking OCPs. Certain OCPs can exacerbate or cause acne. In addition, tetracycline has been reported anecdotally to decrease the efficacy of OCPs, so patients must be counselled.
8. Patients taking chronic antibiotics, especially if using topical antibacterial soaps as well, may develop a gram-negative infection of the face that looks like acne. Lesions must be cultured, and appropriate antibiotic therapy or isotretinoin may be prescribed.

TB

3

Acrodermatitis Chronica Atrophicans and Solitary Lymphocytoma Cutis

Cutaneous Late Lyme Disease

Initial Therapy

Oral tetracycline 500 mg q.i.d. or doxycycline 100 mg b.i.d. for 10–14 days.

Alternative Therapy

1. Oral penicillin V 500 mg q.i.d. for 10–14 days or
2. Intramuscular benzathine penicillin (Bicillin) 1.2–2.4 × 10^6 U weekly for 2–3 weeks, or
3. Oral erythromycin 500 mg q.i.d. (This option is less desirable owing to the low in vitro and in vivo sensitivity of the causative agent to erythromycin.)

Subsequent Therapy

For patients who fail to respond to oral tetracycline and intramuscular benzathine penicillin effective therapies include:

1. Intravenous or intramuscular ceftriaxone 1–2 g q.d. for 14 days, or
2. Intravenous penicillin 20 × 10⁶ U/day for 10 days.

Pitfall

The atrophic lesions of acrodermatitis chronica atrophicans may be permanent.

TB

4

Acrodermatitis Enteropathica

Zinc Deficiency

Zinc deficiency is not only a characteristic of acrodermatitis enteropathica (AE), but also may be associated with nonhealing ulcers, chronic ethanolism, malnutrition, fad diets, and recalcitrant infections. Secondary oral candidiasis (thrush) often complicates AE, and they may need to be treated simultaneously.

Initial Therapy

1. Prescribe oral zinc sulfate 50 mg t.i.d. with meals or fruit juice for children, and doses of up to 800 mg/day for adults for short time periods. Response begins to occur within days.
2. Prescribe oral nystatin 100,000–500,000 U q.i.d. for 2 weeks for *Candida* superinfections and to patients responding slowly to oral zinc alone.

Alternative Therapy

1. Some cases of AE do not clear completely with oral zinc sulfate, presumably because of poor absorption. Amphotericin B lozenges 10 mg q.i.d. for 5 days have been used to increase GI absorption of zinc.
2. Picolinic acid, a chelating agent present in pancreatic secretions, 3–5 tsp/day (6–10 g/day) also has been used to increase zinc absorption.
3. Zinc oxide paste (25% in petrolatum, Lassar's paste), when applied to intertriginous or occluded areas in AE patients, or to ulcers in acquired cases, may improve zinc status locally, leading to improved healing. However, it is unlikely that sufficient absorption occurs for systemic correction of zinc deficiency.

Pitfalls

Hyperzincemia, with zinc toxicity, can result from acute or prolonged overdosing with zinc. Dosages should be adjusted based upon regular (1–2-week) assessment of fasting plasma zinc levels (i.e., before the next oral dose).

PE

5

Actinic Keratosis

Solar Keratosis

Actinic keratoses (AKs) are commonly multiple and occur on chronically sun-exposed areas. Therapy is determined by location (face, scalp, or forearms) and extent (few, multiple). AKs on the lower lip are termed *actinic cheilitis.*

Initial Therapy

FEW LESIONS

Few or solitary lesions on any site are best treated with liquid nitrogen cryotherapy. Extensive lesions may also be managed by repeated cryotherapy.

EXTENSIVE LESIONS

1. Face: Widespread lesions of the face may be treated with applications of 5-fluorouracil (5-FU) 1%–5% cream b.i.d., avoiding the eyelids and naso-labial folds. Expect extensive swelling, erosions, and pain 3–5 days after the start of treatment. Analgesics, including codeine at night, may be required. Continue treatment for at least 2 weeks and occasionally 3–4 weeks, depending on the briskness and severity of the reaction. Application of an intermediate-potency topical steroid for a few days may hasten healing. Complete healing requires an additional month, and a pink flush may be present for up to 3 months.
2. Arms and scalp: The keratoses on these areas tend to be more hypertrophic, so 5-FU 5% is almost always necessary. The lotion formulation, which is stronger, may be necessary. Treatment may need to be continued for 6–8 weeks.
3. Lips: Actinic cheilitis may also be managed with 5-FU 1%–2% cream b.i.d., but the reaction is more severe and more painful than that on the face.

Alternative Therapy

FEW LESIONS

1. Single large (over 1 cm²) AKs may not respond to cryotherapy. After an adequate biopsy, to rule out squamous cell carcinoma, a local course of 5-FU for 2–3 weeks will usually clear the lesion with almost no cosmetic deficit.
2. Hyperkeratotic AKs often require a biopsy for diagnosis and treatment.

EXTENSIVE LESIONS

1. Lesions of the forearms and scalp may not react even to the 5-FU 5% lotion. The addition of tretinoin (Retin A) 0.05%–0.1% cream or Keralyt Gel q.h.s. with 5-FU 5% b.i.d. will usually lead to a brisker and more complete response.
2. Dermabrasion of the scalp may be indicated for extensive AKs not respon-

sive to 5-FU. All but spot dermabrasion should be avoided on the forearm owing to the possibility of scarring. This procedure is rarely required on the face, although a chemical peel (phenol or over 50% trichloracetic acid) may be occasionally useful.

3. Actinic cheilitis is often best managed surgically. The classic surgical approach, a vermilionectomy, involves excision of the whole involved lower lip and a mucosal advancement to close the defect. Laser vaporization of the involved lower lip may become the surgical treatment of choice because of its speed, minimal discomfort, and excellent results.

Subsequent Therapy

1. Outline the cause and natural history of AKs to the patient.
2. Instruct the patient to avoid excess sun exposure and apply a sunscreen daily.
3. In the future chronic application of tretonin may be indicated as a topical chemopreventive agent.
4. See the patient every 6 months and examine the skin carefully for AKs and other cutaneous cancers.

Pitfalls

1. The most serious error is misdiagnosing a basal cell carcinoma or squamous cell carcinoma, with resultant inadequate treatment. In general, routine cryotherapy and topical 5-FU are *not* adequate treatment for cutaneous carcinoma. Although lesions may initially appear to resolve, recurrence is common. The delay in diagnosis may result in more extensive local growth or even metastases. If there is any question, an adequate biopsy prior to therapy is indicated.
2. Cryotherapy may lead to extensive cutaneous necrosis in patients with cryoglobulinemia or cryofibrinogenemia.
3. Hypopigmentation is a common result of overly brisk cryotherapy.
4. Areas treated with 5-FU may become secondarily infected, exaggerating the pain, crusting, and erosions. Systemic antibiotic therapy to cover *S. aureus* is indicated.
5. Contact dermatitis may develop with repeated courses of 5-FU. Pruritus and extension of the erythema and crusts beyond the treated areas are indications of the development of contact dermatitis.
6. While using topical 5-FU patients are photosensitive. Ideally, treatment should be carried out during the winter and patients should avoid sun exposure. Patients usually cannot tolerate the use of sunscreens on areas underoing 5-FU therapy until they heal.

7. Squamous cell carcinomas of the lower lip arising from actinic cheilitis are much more aggressive than those arising from AKs on the rest of the cutaneous surface. Careful follow-up and a high index of suspicion are required when managing lower-lip crusts or ulcerations.

TB

6

Actinomycosis

Initial Therapy

Treatment is with intramuscular penicillin 10–20×10^6 U/day for 3 weeks.

Alternative Therapy

1. For the penicillin-allergic patient, prescribe oral tetracycline or erythromycin 500 mg q.i.d. Total therapy is for 6 months, or 3 months after complete healing, whichever is longer.
2. Amikacin and rifampin may also be useful agents.

Subsquent Therapy

1. It is important to look for underlying bony involvement, especially in the case of cervicofacial actinomycosis. Eradication of an underlying dental source may enhance healing and prevent relapse.
2. After 3 weeks of intravenous penicillin, switch to oral penicillin VK 500 mg q.i.d. with probenecid. Continue therapy for at least 6 months or until the lesion has been stable or has appeared healed for 3 months, whichever is longer. Oral amoxicillin 500 mg q.i.d. may also be used.

Pitfalls

1. Failure to evaluate lesions by appropriate cultures and biopsy often delays diagnosis.

2. Early discontinuation of therapy leads to recurrence.
3. Evaluate the patient for immunosuppression.

TB

7

Alopecia Areata

Alopecia Totalis • Alopecia Universalis

Alopecia areata is characterized by nonscarring hair loss of unknown etiology. Manifestations are most frequently limited to a few oval bald patches. However, a minority of individuals develop extensive areas of hair loss or even loss of all body hair (alopecia totalis or universalis).

Initial Therapy

LIMITED HAIR LOSS

1. No treatment may be required, as regrowth, particularly in alopecia areata, is common in 2–6 months.
2. If treatment is instituted, intralesional injection of corticosteroids may be of value. Inject lesions with triamcinolone 2.5–5 mg/cc, and if necessary repeat treatment every 4–6 weeks. Intralesional corticosteroid injections are not practical for patients with alopecia totalis, but may be used in this setting to induce hair growth in cosmetically important areas such as the eyebrows.

EXTENSIVE HAIR LOSS

1. A reliable, standard initial therapy is not available. (Alternative Therapy, below.)
2. Corticosteroid injections may cause focal reversible scalp depressions.

Alternative Therapy

LIMITED OR EXTENSIVE HAIR LOSS

Multiple modalities have been described, but none is clearly superior.

1. Application of minoxidil 2% or 3% solution q.d. or b.i.d. may be attempted, but efficacy has not been ascertained.
2. Anthralin-induced irritant dermatitis is safe and may be beneficial. Application of anthralin 0.25%–1.0% in petrolatum or paste to the scalp for 20–30 minutes q.d. induces dermatitis. Continue the therapeutic trial for 2–4 months.
3. Contact allergen application may be efficacious. The most frequently studied sensitizer is dichloronitrobenzene (DCNB). Apply DCNB 2% in acetone for sensitization on the forearm initially and follow it with an application of lower concentrations (0.001%–0.1%) to the scalp in an ointment to maintain an eczematous reaction. Response rates are 0%–80%. Use of DCNB therapy is limited by concern about its mutagenicity in bacteria; however, there is no evidence of its occurrence in humans. Squaric acid dibutyl ester, another potent topical allergen that may be used, has the theoretical advantage that it is not a mutagen. Sensitize with a 2% solution in acetone, and elicit dermatitis with a 0.1% solution in acetone.
4. Photochemotherapy (PUVA), using either topically applied or systemic psoralen, may be attempted. Topical solutions (0.1%–0.15%) avoid ocular toxicity.

Pitfalls

1. Corticosteroid injections may cause focal reversible scalp depressions, and has been rarely reported to cause blindness (see Appendix 4).
2. Systemic steroids induce hair growth in patients with extensive alopecia areata, but such therapy is not recommended. High doses are usually required, and hair loss recurs after steroid discontinuation. The complications of long-term high-dose steroid therapy are not justified.
3. Alopecia areata is infrequently associated with other autoimmune disorders, including thyroid disease, vitiligo, pernicious anemia, and Addison's disease.
4. Contact dermatitis therapy may cause widespread dermatitis and lymphadenopathy.
5. Anthralin therapy may cause cutaneous staining (see Ch. 147, Psoriasis).

BW

8

Androgenetic Alopecia

Pattern hair loss occurs in both men and women. The cause is poorly understood, but predisposing factors include inheritance and increased hair follicle sensitivity to androgens.

Therapeutic Alternatives

1. Apply minoxidil 2%–3% in a 40% alcohol and water solution b.i.d. Preliminary information from men with early vertex hair loss indicates acceptable cosmetic hair growth in only one third to one half by 4–8 months. Frontal-bitemporal recession often fails to respond. Therapy must be continued or hair loss recurs. If response is poor or absent, mix minoxidil 3% 50 : 50 with tretinoin 0.01% (Retin-A) and apply b.i.d.
2. Hair transplantation is an excellent therapy in appropriate patients, and can often be combined with surgical scalp reduction. Although simultaneous minoxidil therapy to prevent future hair loss is recommended by some, it is not of proven benefit.
3. Cosmetic techniques, including hair weaving and use of wigs, are useful alternatives.

Pitfalls

1. Do not attempt implantation of artificial hair into the scalp, as foreign-body reactions and scalp infections result.
2. Injection of foreign materials such as paraffin has been attempted in the past, but causes chronic granulomatous reactions and does not grow hair.
3. Injection and topical application of estrogens and progesterones have been attempted, but efficacy is not proven. Injection of estrogens may cause feminization of men.
4. Rule out androgen-excess syndromes in women. They may have adrenal or ovarian cysts or tumors.

BW

9

Angular Cheilitis

Perlèche

Angular cheilitis is due to overgrowth of microorganisms, especially *C. albicans*, at the corners of the mouth. It is seen in five settings: infants; edentulous, usually elderly, persons, owing to constant maceration of the angle of the mouth; adolescents and adults who wear orthodontic devices; diabetics and those who have undergone antibiotic or systemic steroid therapy; and immunosuppressed persons.

Initial Therapy

1. Infants: Oral candidiasis (thrush) is almost always present. Treatment is with oral nystatin suspension (100,000 U/ml) q.i.d., plus application of nystatin ointment to the affected area b.i.d. for 1 week. Excess food and saliva should be carefully washed from the affected area regularly.
2. Elderly edentulous persons: Adjust the dentures, adding vertical dimension. Treat thrush if present. Have the patient clean the denture(s) and apply nystatin ointment or solution to them daily, and apply Mycolog *ointment* or a topical imidazole to the affected area t.i.d. for 2 weeks.
3. Diabetics and post antibiotic/systemic steroid patients: Treat thrush if present. Have the patient apply Mycolog *ointment* or a topical imidazole cream to the perlèche t.i.d. for 2 weeks.
4. Immunosuppressed patients: Treat thrush if present. Have the patient apply Mycolog *ointment* or a topical imidazole cream to the perlèche t.i.d. Topical therapy may need to be maintained if immunosuppression persists.

Alternative Therapy

1. In the elderly, edentulous patient redundant folded skin at the corners of the mouth may predispose to perlèche and may need to be corrected for the perlèche to clear. Collagen injections or surgery may be necessary.
2. Secondary bacterial infection may occur and requires oral antibiotics, as for impetigo.

3. For refractory adult cases prescribe ketoconazole tablets 200 mg b.i.d. for 1–2 weeks.

Pitfalls

1. Evaluation for immunosuppression is indicated if other predisposing factors are not identified.
2. Clotrimazole troches and oral ketoconazole may cause liver function abnormalities.
3. Nystatin and Mycolog ointments, *not* creams, are recommended. They are nonsensitizing. Ointment occlusion of the area prevents maceration and enhances response.
4. If the patient is pruritic, suspect allergic contact dermatitis.
5. Metabolic diseases and deficiencies are rare causes of perlèche.
6. Perlèche, especially when unilateral, that fails to respond as expected may be a sign of a mucocutaneous malignancy.
7. In edentulous and immunosuppressed patients candidiasis may recur very quickly, and preventive therapy consisting of an application of an imidazole cream q.d. may be necessary to prevent recurrences.

TB

10

Aphthous Stomatitis

Canker Sore

Aphthous stomatitis is a frequently recurring disorder of the oral mucous membranes. The diagnosis is made on a clinical basis. Histopathology is not specific. Patients are bothered by lesion symptoms rather than appearance. Because the pathogenesis of this disorder is not understood, rational, highly effective therapy is not available.

Initial Therapy

Initial therapy is symptomatic, and should relieve pain in order to prevent interference with eating.

1. Topical anesthetics: Prescribe a topical anesthetic such as viscous lidocaine 2% (Xylocaine) to be applied directly to aphthae p.r.n. to prevent discomfort. Relief lasts 30–60 minutes.
2. Topical steroids: Prescribe a topical steroid in paste to be applied to lesions 4–6 times/day. The most frequently used is Kenalog in Orabase (triamcinolone 0.1% in gelatin, pectin, carboxymethyl cellulose sodium in Plastibase). Alternative topical steroids of most types have been used without a clear-cut therapeutic advantage. Superpotent steroids in an ointment base (e.g., Temovate, Diprolene) may be used if triamcinolone is ineffective.
3. Systemic steroids: Rarely, mucous membrane pain is so severe as to interfere with nutrition or prevent sleep. In such patients, intramuscular Kenalog 40–60 mg/day may be necessary to control symptoms. Systemic therapy should be accompanied by the topical measures outlined above.

Alternative Therapy

Multiple recurrences, or chronic, symptomatic aphthous ulcers, are particularly difficult to manage. Multiple unproven therapies have been attempted in such cases. These include:

1. Hematinics: Recurrent oral aphthoses may respond to correction of underlying hematologic abnormalities. Replacement therapy has included administration of iron, vitamin B_{12}, or folic acid.
2. Tetracycline: Tetracycline suspension (250 mg/5 ml q.i.d.) may be used as a 2-minute mouthwash. Although incidence or recurrence is not affected, some believe that duration and severity of symptoms may be reduced.
3. Gluten-free diet: This approach may be worthwhile in recalcitrant cases.

Pitfalls

Although most recurrent oral aphthae are not associated with underlying medical problems, they may be the sole manifestation of pernicious anemia, folic acid or iron deficiency, celiac disease, regional enteritis, Behcet's syndrome or familial malabsorption of vitamin B$_{12}$. In addition, other diagnostic possibilities, such as viral illnesses, pemphigus, pemphigoid, and erythema multiforme, may be sought and ruled out by biopsy.

BW

11

Appendigeal Tumors

Adnexal Tumors

Both benign and malignant tumors may arise from the cutaneous adnexa (hair follicles, sweat glands, and sebaceous glands).

Initial Therapy

1. A biopsy is usually necessary to establish the diagnosis, except for syringomas.
2. Surgical therapy is the only available alternative in most cases, but is only required for malignant or locally aggressive lesions, or when requested by the patient for cosmetic reasons.
3. Eccrine hidrocystomas may occasionally be controlled by application of topical atropine 2% in petrolatum b.i.d.

Pitfall

In some cases the pathologic interpretation of adnexal tumors may be difficult and their biologic behavior hard to predict. Consider referral or consultation.

TB

12

Atopic Dermatitis, Adult

Therapy of adult atopic dermatitis may be approached as management of either acute, subacute, or chronic dermatitis. In addition, therapy should be based on the extent of skin involvement (i.e., generalized vs. localized disease).

Initial Therapy

1. Hydration and debridement: Prescribe oilated colloidal oatmeal (Aveeno) baths (1/2 cup/bath) b.i.d. Instruct the patient to use cool-to-tepid water, soak 15–20 minutes, and gently pat dry with a soft towel.
2. Suppression of inflammation: Prescribe high-potency, fluorinated steroids (*cream* during acute phase, both for drying effect and to avoid occlusion of infected lesions) to be applied after the bath. A thin film should be applied to the rash only b.i.d.
3. Suppression of pruritus: Give oral antihistamines (hydroxyzine, initially 10 mg q.i.d., increasing to 50 mg q.i.d. until pruritus is suppressed, or until specific side effects limit dosage). At *bedtime* diphenhydramine (Benadryl) 50–100 mg may be substituted for hydroxyzine for its additional sedative effect.

Ancillary Therapy

1. Treatment of secondary infection: Colonization with *S. aureus* is common, although often inapparent. Thus, even in the absence of obvious infection, treat patients with acute dermatitis who have tenderness, crusts, and/or oozing empirically with erythromycin or a semisynthetic penicillin (e.g., dicloxacillin 1 g/day for 7–10 days). In patients with recurrent infections, obtain cultures and sensitivities first to ensure that resistant organisms have not established themselves.
2. General measures: Advise the patient to cut nails; use mild soaps (e.g., Dove; avoid Ivory) and soapless cleansers (e.g., Cetaphil); avoid wool and acrylic clothing; and avoid bathing more often than once a day, especially during winter months. Soap need be applied only to intertriginous sites (groin and axillae).

Subsequent Therapy (after rash abates, usually in 7–10 days)

1. Hydration: Continue oilated colloidal oatmeal baths.
2. Suppression of inflammation: Switch from a cream to an ointment formulation of an intermediate potency topical steroid (see Appendix 1) (e.g., triamcinolone 0.1% or betamethasone valerate 0.1%), which is applied b.i.d.
3. Suppression of pruritus: Continue antihistamines at maximum tolerated dosage indefinitely.
4. In addition to the steroid therapy, emolliate the entire skin surface (except the face) with a water-in-oil (ointment) preparation (e.g., petrolatum (Vaseline), Nivea, or aquaphor (Eucerin)). *Note:* Lotions or creams can exacerbate underlying dry skin conditions.
5. Other measures:
   a. UVB is helpful in further reducing inflammation, and can be obtained from natural sunlight; encourage exposure between the hours of 11:00 and 2:00 during March through October. Fair-skinned individuals should avoid sunburn—even short exposures are beneficial.
   b. Artificial UVB: Give 2–5 treatments/week, gradually increasing exposure times.
   c. Photochemotherapy (PUVA) is highly effective and requires fewer treatments than psoriasis, but is controversial because of possible long-term side effects.
   d. Tar (with or without UVB): T/Derm (Neutrogena) or Fototar (Elder) are two nondrying, cosmetically acceptable tar preparations that can be applied q.d. or b.i.d. with the purpose of inducing remissions; potentiating UVB; and reducing steroid requirements (fewer side effects and lower cost).
   e. Sytemic steroids: See Pitfalls.
   f. Use of a cool-air humidifier in the home during the months of October–March is very helpful for severe, recalcitrant cases.
   g. Evening primrose oil, because of its high content of γ-linolenic acid, appears to help some patients with severe atopic dermatitis. Doses of 6 g/day or more are required.
   h. Measures of unproven benefit: Dietary modifications, despite an extensive literature, are of unproven value; allergy testing (scratch testing), followed by exclusion of offending allergens, also is not generally helpful.

Pitfalls

1. As noted above, colonization with *S. aureus* is common, often inapparent, and is often the trigger for fresh exacerbations of disease.

2. Atopic dermatitis tends to flare during the winter months unless the measures described under Subsequent Therapy are continued indefinitely.

3. Two precautions should be discussed with patients using oilated colloidal oatmeal: first, it can clog plumbing, and second, it is mandatory to use a rubber bath mat to avoid slipping in the tub.

4. Although antihistamines can be sedating, tachyphylaxis to the soporific effects occurs within a few days, allowing higher and higher doses, if necessary. Initially, however, patients must be warned about the risks of operating motor vehicles and additive sedation from alcohol intake.

5. Systemic steroids are not generally necessary, and should be avoided in atopic dermatitis. Although they are extremely effective, patients tend to become overly dependent, and side effects of chronic steroid therapy can result.

PE

13

Atopic Dermatitis, Juvenile

Childhood atopic dermatitis can present as acute, subacute, or chronic dermatitis, and disease can vary from a localized to a generalized disease process. The intensity of therapy should be appropriate for the severity of patient presentation.

Initial Therapy

1. Hydration and debridement: Prescribe oilated colloidal oatmeal (Aveeno) baths (1/2 cup/bath) q.d. (b.i.d. for severe cases). Instruct the patient to use cool-to-tepid water, soak 15–20 minutes, and gently pat dry with a soft towel.

2. Suppression of inflammation: For acute or subacute dermatitis, after bathing, and at one other time (b.i.d.), a thin film of low potency, nonfluorinated steroid *cream* (e.g., desonide or hydrocortisone 2.5%, see Appendix 1) is applied to the rash only. For chronic dermatitis, a comparable-potency preparation in an *ointment* formulation is used. In acute atopic dermatitis, after the rash begins to improve, switch from a cream to an ointment formulation.

3. Suppression of pruritus: Administer hydroxyzine syrup, initially 5–10 mg q.i.d., increasing the dose as tolerated, until pruritus is suppressed. Alternatively, administer diphenhydramine elixir (Benadryl) 12.5–25 mg q.i.d., increasing as tolerated. *Note:* About 20%–25% of children will experience paradoxical hyperactivity with either hydroxyzine or diphenhydramine. Fortunately, in almost all such cases the other antihistamines will not elicit a comparable response.

Ancillary Therapy

1. Superinfection with *S. aureus* is common, although often inapparent. Thus, even in the absence of obvious infection, treat patients with acute dermatitis who have tenderness, crusts, and/or oozing empirically with erythromycin or a semisynthetic penicillin (usually dicloxacillin 25 mg/kg/day for 7 days). In patients with recurrent infections, obtain cultures and sensitivities first to ensure that resistant organisms are not present.
2. General measures: Instruct the patient to cut nails, use mild soaps (avoiding Ivory), and avoid wool or acrylic clothing (cotton is best).
3. Avoid systemic steroids (see Pitfalls).

Subsequent Therapy (after rash abates, usually in 7–10 days):

1. Hydration: Continue cool, oilated oatmeal baths and use of mild soaps.
2. Suppression of inflammation: Prescribe a low-potency steroid ointment to be applied b.i.d. to the residual rash only. Steroids can be stopped when the rash is gone, but other measures must be continued or a relapse is likely.
3. Suppression of pruritus: Continue antihistamines at maximum tolerated dose throughout the high-risk season (October–March).
4. The entire skin surface (except the face) should be emolliated with a water-in-oil (ointment) preparation (e.g., aquaphor (Eucerin)) q.d. after bathing while skin is still damp. *Note:* Use of "dry skin" lotions and creams can have a deleterious, drying effect on atopic skin.
5. Other measures:
   a. Naturally occurring UVB, available only between the hours of 11:00 and 2:00 from March to October at northern latitudes, provides useful, ancillary anti-inflammatory activity.
   b. Use of a cool-air humidifier in the bedroom between October and March is very helpful in stubborn, recalcitrant cases because it creates summertime humidities during winter months.
   c. Evening primrose oil, a γ-linolenic acid-enriched preparation, reportedly helps some children with refractory atopic dermatitis.

d. Neither dietary modifications nor allergy (scratch) testing, with subsequent exclusion of offending allergens, is required in the management of patients with atopic dermatitis. In several refractory cases careful trials of elimination diets (for 6–8-week periods) followed by reintroduction of the eliminated foods and the evaluation by means of a symptom diary is the most effective way to evaluate for a potential exacerbating food allergen. RAST and prick tests do not reliably identify children who may have food allergy. Foods to be eliminated are eggs, nuts (including peanuts), cow's milk, wheat, fish, and soy. Sequential elimination diets are required, a painstaking process for the parent and often of low yield (1%–20%).

Pitfalls

1. As noted above, acute atopic dermatitis is commonly colonized with *S. aureus*, often inapparently, and frequently infection may trigger subsequent disease exacerbations.
2. After recurrent courses of antibiotics, *S. aureus* resistant to semisynthetic penicillins and/or erythromycin can emerge. Some alternate antibiotics, such as clindamycin and trimethoprim-sulfamethoxazole, remain alternative possibilities in such cases.
3. Atopic dermatitis tends to flare during winter months unless the measures described under Subsequent Therapy are continued indefinitely.
4. As noted above, paradoxical agitation and/or hyperactivity can complicate therapy with antihistamines in children.
5. Bath oils and powders such as oilated colloidal oatmeal can clog plumbing and cause serious falls in the bathtub. To minimize the likelihood of the latter, a rubber bath mat should be used.
6. Systemic steroids are not generally necessary, and should be avoided in atopic dermatitis. Although they are extremely effective, patients tend to become overly dependent, and side effects of chronic steroid therapy can result.

PE

14

Atrophie Blanche

Livedoid Vasculitis • Segmental Hyalinizing Vasculitis • Summer/Winter Ulcerations

Atrophie blanche is not a distinct entity, but is probably the end stage of livedoid vasculitis. Therapy is most frequently aimed at healing the resultant ankle ulceration and at treating the primary disorder causing the vascular damage.

Therapy of Ankle Ulceration

Therapeutic alternatives are identical to those described for cutaneous ulcers (see Ch. 41).

Initial Therapy of Livedoid Vasculitis

The therapeutic prevention of additional vascular lesions is the therapeutic goal. No systemic approach has been universally successful, and this disorder is notoriously difficult to treat. The following agents have been employed with varying success:

1. Agents that inhibit platelet function: Treatment is with aspirin 325 mg b.i.d. and dipyridamole (Persantine) 50–75 mg t.i.d. to q.i.d. for 2–8 months.
2. Vasodilators: The following have been employed and may be useful.
    a. Nifedipine, a calcium channel blocker, 10 mg t.i.d. for 6 months.
    b. Guanethidine 10 mg b.i.d. to q.i.d.
    c. Nicotinic acid 100 mg t.i.d.
3. Enhancement of cutaneous blood flow: Treat with pentoxifylline (Trental) 400 mg t.i.d. for at least 2–3 months.
4. Anticoagulants: Subcutaneous heparin 5,000 U q.3d. for at least 3 months.
5. Fibrinolysis therapy: Phenformin 50 mg b.i.d. and ethyl estrinol 2–6

mg/day have been used, although Phenformin is no longer available in the United States.

6. Sulfones: Sulfapyridine 500 mg–4 g/day and dapsone 50–200 mg/day have been used with variable results.

7. Systemic steroids: Prednisone 40–60 mg/day has been useful.

Subsequent Therapy of Livedoid Vasculitis

In general, treat patients until the ankle ulcer resolves; treatment may be reinstituted in the event of recurrent painful ulceration.

Pitfalls

1. The therapist must be concerned with potential side effects of the various drugs used in treating this disease.

2. Proper diagnosis of ankle ulceration is important. Ulcers may result from a variety of conditions, such as venous stasis, arterial insufficiency, cholesterol emboli, and other forms of small vessel vasculitis, which do not require the use of the agents listed above.

BW

15

Atypical Mycobacteria

Although several mycobacterial organisms have been associated with skin lesions, only two, *M. ulcerans* and *M. marinum*, are common pathogens, with the latter by far the most common agent in nontropical countries.

M. MARINUM

Initial Therapy

1. Once the diagnosis is established, minocycline 100 mg b.i.d. for 2 months is usually curative for cases with multiple lesions.

2. Excisional surgery or curettage and desiccation is curative for small lesions or limited numbers of lesions of *M. marinum*.

Alternative Therapy

1. For patients who experience unacceptable CNS side effects from minocycline, tetracycline, 1 g b.i.d. is almost as effective, but less convenient.
2. Trimethoprim-sulfamethoxazole (Bactrim DS or Septra DS) 1 tablet/day (equivalent to 160 mg trimethoprim/800 mg sulfamethoxazole) for 2–3 months is also effective.
3. Rifampicin and/or ethambutol reportedly are also effective, but remain the third choice after tetracycline or trimethoprim-sulfamethoxazole.
4. Radiation therapy can shrink large lesions. Usually 12 treatments of 150 rads each are required.

M. ULCERANS

Initial Therapy

Clofazimine 100 mg b.i.d. for 1 month, with excisional surgery, is the only known effective therapy.

Pitfalls

1. Mycobacterial infections can appear sporotrichoid; hence, biopsies from patients with this pattern should be examined and cultured for both mycobacteria and deep fungi.
2. Minocycline can produce vertigo, dizziness, and/or headaches (with or without signs of increased CNS pressure), especially in those receiving doses of 100 mg b.i.d. (i.e., up to 10% of patients). Ingestion with meals can reduce dizziness, but the drug should be stopped if symptoms persist.
3. Rarely, *M. marinum* infections produce concurrent synovitis, arthritis, and/or osteomyelitis.
4. Scarring, lymphedema, and contractures can follow extensive atypical mycobacterial infections.

PE

16

Balanitis

Balanitis is a nonspecific term meaning inflammation of the glans penis. It is most commonly multifactorial in etiology, restricted to the uncircumcised, and presents as a mildly symptomatic scaly, red macule or patch. Acute suppurative balanitis may also occur in the uncircumcised. The therapy of those two types is discussed separately. Certain specific skin diseases (e.g., Reiter's disease, psoriasis, lichen planus, lichen sclerosis et atrophicus, syphilis, and scabies) may affect the glans penis preferentially. A total skin examination to rule out these other conditions should be performed. Any area of balanitis not responding to conventional therapy should be biopsied to rule out carcinoma in situ (erythroplasia).

ERYTHEMATOUS SCALY PATCH TYPE

Initial Therapy

1. Counsel the patient on the pathogenesis (moisture, bacterial and candidal overgrowth, and if appropriate, inadequate local hygiene).
2. Instruct the patient to retract the foreskin and wash with a mild soap (rinsed off well) b.i.d.
3. Prescribe an imidazole cream to be applied sparingly to the area after washing.
4. Order a serologic test for syphilis and evaluate the patient for diabetes mellitus.
5. Evaluate the sexual partner(s) for candidal, bacterial, or trichomonal vaginitis, proctitis, and oral thrush.

Alternative Therapy

Iodochlorhydroxyquin (Vioform) may be used instead of an imidazole cream.

Subsequent Therapy

1. A mild topical steroid hydrocortisone (0.5% to 2.5%) may be added to the topical imidazole in refractory cases.
2. Take a careful drug history to rule out a fixed drug eruption. Consider the rare possibility of an allergic contact dermatitis (e.g., from condoms or vaginal hygiene spray).
3. Biopsy patients not responding to these measures.
4. Circumcision will usually result in resolution in refractory cases.

Pitfalls

1. Do not make the diagnosis of a nonspecific balanitis until other skin diseases, including carcinoma in situ, have been ruled out.
2. Do not refer a patient for circumcision until a biopsy has been performed.
3. Avoid prolonged steroid use on the glans penis, as atrophy is common. In addition, the withdrawal of topical steroids when they have been used chronically often results in a flare of symptoms. Steroid dependency becomes a problem.

ACUTE SUPPURATIVE BALANITIS

Initial Therapy

1. If the foreskin cannot be retracted, consider referral to a urologist for a dorsal slit.
2. Perform a bacterial culture of the purulent discharge.
3. Evaluate the patient for urethritis, especially gonococcal, candidal, or trichomonal.
4. Order a serologic test for syphilis.
5. Instruct the patient to retract the foreskin b.i.d. and gently compress with Burow's solution 1 : 20 with acetic acid 0.25% for 15 minutes.
6. Prescribe an imidazole cream to be applied b.i.d. after compressing.

Subsequent Therapy

1. If the bacterial culture grows a single pathogen (other than *P. aeruginosa*) and the balanitis persists, treat with an appropriate oral antibiotic. If *P. aeruginosa* is cultured, prescribe gentamycin ophthalmic ointment to be applied b.i.d. If an anaerobe or *Bacteroides* sp. are cultured, prescribe metronidazole 500 mg b.i.d. for 5 days.

2. Evaluate the patient for diabetes mellitus.
3. Take a careful history of intermittent drug ingestion to rule out a fixed drug eruption.
4. Evaluate the sexual partner(s) for infection with *C. albicans*, *T. vaginalis*, and *G. vaginalis*.

Pitfall

Failure to retract the foreskin and carefully examine the patient for a penile ulcer or urethritis will often lead to a misdiagnosis.

TB

17

Basal Cell Carcinoma

Basal cell carcinomas (BCCs) are best managed by persons expert in their recognition, natural history, and treatment. Failure to correctly manage tumors initially may lead to significant cosmetic deformity. General guidelines are given below, but the correct choice of therapy for individual lesions depends on age, sex, location, pigmentary type, and history of prior treatment. A biopsy to confirm the diagnosis should, in general, be performed before treating any lesion.

Initial Therapy

1. Surgical excision with a 2–5-mm margin of normal tissue is usually optimal. Send the specimen for pathologic evaluation for adequacy of excision.
2. In elderly persons (over 60 years) and in the debilitated, radiation therapy provides excellent results. It is also excellent for surgically complex lesions.
3. For superficial or small (under 1 cm) lesions of the trunk, curettage and desiccation (C & D) provides an acceptable cure rate and good cosmesis. C & D scars may be unsightly, and so this is not the preferred treatment for facial lesions.
4. Facial lesions over 1 cm in diameter that have been present for more than 2 years and lesions located in the temple, eyelid, medial canthus, nose, and nasolabial fold are more likely to recur. Consider them as potential candi-

dates for micrographic surgery (Moh's chemosurgery). In these cases surgical excision or radiation therapy is preferred, and C & D, in general, not recommended.

5. All recurrent BCCs, BCCs whose margins are indistinct, morpheaform BCCs, and tumors that will require extensive reconstruction to repair the surgical defect are appropriately managed by micrographic surgery.

Alternative Therapy

For the rare patient unable to tolerate radiation therapy or surgery, local cryotherapy with thermocouple control may be an excellent alternative.

Subsequent Therapy

1. Patient education with respect to pathogenesis and natural hsitory of basal cell carcinomas is essential. Sun protection must be stressed.
2. Perform a complete examination of all sun-exposed skin on the initial visit and once yearly thereafter.

Pitfall

Failure to correctly diagnose and treat BCCs may lead to additional scarring or cosmetic deformity. A biopsy of any suspicious lesion is required.

TB

18

Basal Cell Nevus Syndrome

Initial Therapy

1. Surgical excision of all tumors is the best therapy and is performed if possible. Follow the guidelines for the management of routine basal cell carcinomas (see Ch. 17). Radiation therapy is relatively contraindicated.

2. Genetic counselling and examination of family members is important.
3. Strict sun protection (avoidance) must be stressed.
4. Evaluate the patient for associated conditions, especially jaw cysts.

Subsequent Therapy

Although the synthetic retinoids are *not* currently useful for chemotherapy, they may be used in chemoprevention. In patients developing multiple new lesions, low doses of these agents may be given with informed consent. (Apparently therapy must be lifelong.) Chronic toxicity, especially skeletal, has limited the effectiveness of the retinoids.

Pitfalls

1. Do not underestimate the potential for cosmetic disfigurement. Attempt to identify lesions early and eradicate each one completely.
2. Retinoids should only be used by physicians experienced with these agents and their potential side effects. Full informed consent is essential. Childbearing is absolutely contraindicated.
3. Because many of these patients are young, avoid radiation therapy.

TB

19

Behçet Syndrome

Behçet syndrome is a disorder of unknown cause characterized in most severe cases by fever, neurologic abnormalities, oral and genital mucous membrane ulceration, and associated uveitis. Therapy is notoriously difficult, but should be aimed at relief of cutaneous symptoms and prevention of blindness.

SYSTEMIC THERAPY

Initial Therapy

For severely affected patients, begin therapy with prednisone 1 mg/kg/day in a single or divided dose, and azathioprine 100–200 mg/day. Expect clinical response within 3–5 weeks.

Subsequent Therapy

After resolution of ophthalmic and cutaneous lesions, taper steroids by 10 mg each week to the lowest q.o.d. dose that maintains clinical remission. When possible, discontinue azathioprine and treat with low-dose systemic steroids alone.

Alternative Therapy

1. Chlorambucil 0.1–0.2 mg/kg/day, tapered to 2 mg/day, may be used instead of azathioprine. Some prefer this agent; however, the side effects of sterility and chromosomal damage limit its use.
2. Cyclosporin 10 mg/kg/day has been successfully employed, but its use is limited by renal toxicity.
3. If available, thalidomide 200 mg b.i.d. for 5 days, tapered to 100 mg b.i.d. for 1–2 months is an alternative with apparent efficacy. Thalidomide is a known teratogen; caution premenopausal women about its teratogenic effects and perform a pregnancy test before beginning therapy with thalidomide. Thalidomide is only available in the U.S. through the Food and Drug Administration.

Unproven Alternatives Therapy

Multiple unproven agents have been used in a few patients who do not respond to the above alternatives. These include:

1. Dapsone 100 mg/day.
2. Colchicine 0.5 mg b.i.d. or t.i.d.
3. Acyclovir 400 mg q.4h.
4. Ketoconazole 200–400 mg/day.

TOPICAL THERAPY

Initial Therapy

Topical cutaneous therapy is aimed at control of symptoms and is generally identical to that employed for therapy of aphthous ulceration (see Ch. 11).

BW

20

Black Hairy Tongue

Initial Therapy

Daily brushing of the tongue with a toothbrush will usually reduce the color and filamentous hyperkeratosis.

Ancillary Therapy

A 40% solution of urea in water may be applied to the tongue for several minutes prior to brushing for additional benefit.

TB

21

Bowen's Disease

Squamous Cell Carcinoma in Situ

Initial Therapy

Complete surgical excision is the preferred therapy when feasible. This may require staged excision.

Alternative Therapy

1. For frail patients or lesions not easily excised, radiation therapy may be used. It should be restricted to patients over 60 years.
2. Cryotherapy, as done for other cutaneous carcinomas, may be curative.
3. Application of topical 5-fluorouracil 5% cream b.i.d for 6 weeks has been recommended. Because Bowen's disease extends down the hair follicle, this therapy may have a higher recurrence rate.

Pitfalls

1. Although a small biopsy from a large lesion may reveal Bowen's disease, invasive squamous cell carcinoma may be present in another part of the lesion. Therapies not involving pathologic review may miss this and lead to inadequate therapy.
2. Bowen's disease may occur in non-sun-exposed areas.
3. Bowenoid papulosis of the genitalia caused by infection with human papilloma virus type 16 may mimic Bowen's disease histologically. (See Ch. 185, Warts.)

TB

22

Bullous Pemphigoid

Bullous pemphigoid is a benign, usually self-limited inflammatory subepidermal blistering disorder of the elderly. The initial goal of therapy is to control itching and reduce blister formation to a level consistent with individual patient comfort.

Initial Therapy

Treat with oral prednisone alone at 40–60 mg/day in a single morning dose. A dramatic clinical response will be seen in 70–80% of patients after 2–3 weeks.

Subsequent Therapy

After 2–3 weeks, reduce prednisone to 30 mg/day by reduction of the daily dose by 10 mg/week. Then, over the next 2–3 weeks, reduce prednisone to 30 mg q.o.d. Finally, decrease the q.o.d. dose of prednisone by 5 mg/week. When 10 mg q.o.d. is reached, taper dose by 1 mg q.o.d. each week until the lowest amount of prednisone consistent with therapeutic goals is reached.

Alternative Therapy

Alternative agents may be used in patients who do not rapidly respond to systemic steroids or in patients in whom the use of systemic steroids is contraindicated.

1. If the patient responds poorly to prednisone, has persistent severe disease and if clinical response is not achieved after 3 weeks, begin an immunosuppressive agent in combination with prednisone. Alternatives include:
   a. Azathioprine (Imuran) 100–150 mg/day. When clinical response is noted (within 2–4 weeks), taper azathioprine and prednisone until the patient is taking prednisone alone.
   b. Cyclophosphamide (Cytoxan) 100–150 mg/day.
   c. Methotrexate 2.5–15 mg p.o. 2×/week to q.o.d.
2. A variety of agents may be employed in patients with severe osteoporosis,

severe hypertension, or diabetes:
  a. Erythromycin 500 mg q.i.d. or tetracycline 500 mg q.i.d. plus niacin-amide 50–250 mg/day have been used for their anti-inflammatory action.
  b. Dapsone 50–200 mg/day.
  c. Cyclosporin 6–10 mg/day.
  d. Plasmapheresis to remove circulating pemphigoid antibody may be of value, but should be combined with cyclophosphamide 50–150 mg to inhibit antibody production.

Pitfalls

The major pitfalls in bullous pemphigoid therapy include overly aggressive therapy with systemic steroids, complications of improperly used steroids and immunosuppressives, and incorrect diagnosis.

1. Bullous pemphigoid is self-limited, and is *not* life-threatening. Complete suppression of blister formation is not essential. Therefore, do not increase systemic steroids in responding patients whose blister formation is not completely stopped. The use of high-potency topical steroids on locally occurring lesions may be of value in such patients.
2. Potential complications of systemic steroids and immunosuppressants must be carefully sought in all patients so treated (see Appendix 5).
3. Other bullous diseases such as epidermolysis bullosa acquisita, erythema multiforme, and bullous drug eruptions may clinically resemble pemphigoid, and may explain atypical therapeutic responses.

BW

23

Bullous Systemic Lupus Erythematosus

Although bullous systemic lupus erythematosus (bullous SLE) and epidermolysis bullosa acquisita (see Ch. 55) are immunopathologically similar, their clinical behavior is different. Bullous SLE usually responds to therapy.

Initial Therapy

1. Evaluate the patient for SLE and treat appropriately for any complications of this disorder (see Ch. 169). The appearance of bullae in SLE is often *not* associated with a flare of the underlying SLE.
2. Dapsone 50–200 mg/day usually leads to a rapid resolution of the bullous lesions.
3. Stress the importance of sun protection and the daily use of a broad-spectrum sunscreen of SPF 15 or greater.

Pitfalls

The most common side effects of dapsone therapy are hemolysis and a hypersensitivity syndrome (see Ch. 84, Hansen's Disease).

TB

24

Cellulitis

Cellulitis can occur as a primary disease entity or it can complicate a pre-existing dermatosis (i.e., microbes may enter the skin via either an inapparent or an obvious portal of entry). The choice of parenteral vs. oral therapy is influenced by the co-existence of fever, leukocytosis, and/or lymphangitis, and by the location of the infection (e.g., classic erysipelas of the face, periorbital cellulitis, or cellulitis that complicates pre-existing lymphedema of the lower extremities mandates parenteral therapy). Although initial therapy is dictated by the likelihood that the causative organisms are streptococci, in children *H. influenza* is a fairly common cause of facial cellulitis, and in immuno-compromised individuals almost any organism(s) may be responsible. Finally, early in their course, more serious soft tissue infections, such as necrotizing fasciitis, can resemble cellulitis.

MANAGEMENT OF UNCOMPLICATED CELLULITIS

Initial Therapy

1. In the absence of material for Gram stain or culture and absolute diagnostic criteria, direct therapy against both coagulase-positive *S. aureus* and *S. pyogenes*.
2. Treat with oral dicloxacillin 500 mg q.i.d. for 10 days or oral cephalexin 500 mg q.i.d. for 10 days (penicillin-allergic individuals should be monitored initially for possible cross-reactivity).

Alternative Therapy

1. Erythromycin 500 mg q.i.d. for 10 days.
2. Ciprofloxacin 500 mg b.i.d. for 10 days; for severe, complicated infections, 750 mg q.12h. until a response occurs, followed by reduction to 500 mg b.i.d. until the patient is clear of disease. The latter agent may be the drug of choice for methicillin-resistant staphylococci and penicillin-allergic individuals in whom bacteriocidal antibiotics are indicated (e.g., immuno-suppressed, HIV-positive, and other chronically ill patients). *Note:* Ciprofloxacin and other quinoline antibiotics are contraindicated in the pediatric age group and in pregnancy, and are not as effective as the other classes of antibiotics for the treatment of pure streptococcal or anaerobic infections.

Ancillary Therapy

During first 24–48 hours (i.e., until signs of infection diminish dramatically):

1. *Warm compresses* should be applied b.i.d. or t.i.d. for 20–30 minutes. *Note:* Avoid *hot* compresses, which can induce hemorrhagic bullae over streptococcal cellulitis.
2. Infected, dependent extremities should be elevated.
3. In the presence of substantial discomfort mild analgesics (e.g., acetaminophen with codeine 0.5 q.4h. p.r.n. pain) may be given.

Subsequent Therapy

1. Successfully treated cellulitis should begin to respond to the above therapy within 48 hours. Failure to respond promptly may indicate infection by an

antibiotic-resistant strain or an unusual organism. If cultures and sensitivities have been obtained, adjust therapy accordingly (see Alternative Therapy, above).

2. Regardless of promptness of response, continue therapy for the full course to prevent both emergence of resistant strains and recurrent infections.

3. In cellulitis secondary to a pre-existing dermatosis treat the primary disease to eliminate the "portal of entry" (see appropriate chapters).

Pitfalls

1. Cultures and Gram stains often cannot be obtained, and clinical criteria do not distinguish reliably between cellulitis owing to staphylococci and that owing to streptococci. Hence, initial coverage should be directed at both.

2. An increasing number of staphylococcal isolates are resistant to semisynthetic penicillins, cephalosporins, and erythromycin.

3. Failure to respond promptly to appropriate antibiotic therapy should raise other diagnostic possibilities (e.g., an unusual organism, panniculitis, or superficial thrombophlebitis).

4. Infections commonly recur when the full course of therapy has not been completed.

5. Patients with diabetes mellitus or decubitus ulcers should be managed as having complicated cellulitis (see below).

MANAGEMENT OF COMPLICATED CELLULITIS

Patients with systemic symptoms, cellulitis of the face (erysipelas), decubitus ulcers, diabetes mellitus, or dependent extremities should be hospitalized initially, as parenteral therapy is needed either to prevent sepsis or to deliver sufficient tissue levels of drug (e.g., to a lymphedematous extremity).

Initial Therapy

1. Treat against both staphylococci and streptococci, unless Gram stains or cultures can be obtained.

2. Administer oxacillin or nafcillin 1.5–3 gr q.4h. for 48–72 hours, followed by oral therapy as described above (in the non-penicillin-allergic individual).

3. Add aminoglycosides to the initial therapeutic regimen for patients with either diabetes or decubiti who are septic.

4. Intravenous vancomycin, clindamycin, or cephalosporins can be administered to penicillin-allergic individuals.
5. Clindamycin may be preferred to penicillins in patients with decubiti penicillinase-resistant infection because of the added risk of anaerobic infection.
6. In documented streptococcal infection, optimal therapy comprises aqueous penicillin G 12–16 gr/day continuous intravenous infusion for 48–72 hours followed by oral penicillin VK 500 mg q.i.d. for a total of 10 days.

Ancillary Therapy

Include warm compresses, elevation, and analgesics, as described above.

Subsequent Therapy

1. Successfully treated, complicated cellulitis should demonstrate a response to parenteral antibiotics within 48 hours. After a satisfactory response, the patient can be switched to oral antibiotics for the remainder of the treatment course, which generally can be accomplished on an outpatient basis. Failure to respond promptly may indicate the presence of an antibiotic-resistant strain, and alternative therapies (see above) should be implemented (dictated wherever possible by culture and sensitivities).
2. Failure to respond promptly also should alert physicians to other, more serious diagnostic possibilities (e.g., necrotizing fasciitis).
3. In cellulitis secondary to a pre-existing dermatosis, therapy should be directed against the primary disease to eliminate the "portal of entry."
4. In cellulitis arising within a chronically lymphadematous extremity, prolonged parenteral and oral antibiotic therapy (14–21 days) often is required to produce clearing. Patients with a history of frequent recurrences may be candidates for long-term, prophylactic oral antibiotic therapy (penicillin VK or erythromycin 250 mg/day).

Pitfalls

1. Evaluate patients with systemic symptoms for possible bacteremia, septicemia, and/or endocarditis.
2. Cellulitis can mask an underlying osteomyelitis, or it can progress to involve the periosteum.
3. As described above, be aware of the possibility of antibiotic-resistant staphylococcal strains, as well as more serious infections (see Subsequent Therapy, above).

4. Streptococcal infections respond more slowly to semisynthetic penicillins and cephalosporins than to plain penicillin. Manage documented streptococcal infections with aqueous and oral penicillin.
5. Recurrences are common in patients with chronic lymphedema. Therefore, consider prophylactic oral antibiotics and aggressive management of lymphedema.

PE

25

Chancroid

The diagnosis of chancroid is largely clinical, although improved culture techniques allow isolation of the causative organism, *H. ducreyi.*

Initial Therapy

1. Oral erythromycin 500 mg q.i.d. for 7 days, or
2. Intramuscular ceftriaxone 250 mg in a single dose.

Alternative Therapy

1. Trimethoprim-sulfamethoxazole 160–800 mg (1 double-dose or 2 single-dose tablets) b.i.d. for at least 7 days, or
2. Trimethoprim-sulfamethoxazole 640–3200 mg (4 double-dose or 8 single-dose tablets) at one time, or
3. Augmentin (amoxicillin 500 mg and potassium clavulanate 125 mg) t.i.d. for 7 days.

Subsequent Therapy

1. Successfully treated ulcers will show evidence of healing by 7 days.
2. Inguinal nodes (buboes) may continue to progress despite adequate treatment. Aspirate fluctuant nodes with a large-bore needle.
3. Evaluate all patients for other STDs.
4. Sexual contacts of infected persons must be traced and treated.

Pitfalls

1. The antimicrobial sensitivity of *H. ducreyi* is constantly changing; direct therapy by antimicrobial sensitivity tests on the isolated strain, or by known antibiotic sensitivity patterns in the community of acquisition.
2. Look for simultaneous infection in the lesion by herpes simplex and/or syphilis.
3. Gram stains are not always diagnostically reliable.

TB

26

Cheilitis Granulomatosa

Melkersson–Rosenthal Syndrome

Initial Therapy

Treat with intralesional triamcinolone acetonide 10 mg/cc to the affected lip.

Alternative Therapy

Prescribe oral prednisone 40–60 mg/day for 2–3 weeks, then taper the dose.

Subsequent Therapy

1. Search for underlying dental or sinus inflammation. The treatment of these hidden foci of infection may lead to improvement of the cheilitis.
2. Crohn's disease may present as a granulomatous cheilitis, therefore a GI evaluation is indicated.
3. If intralesional steroids have led to improvement, they usually may need to be repeated at monthly intervals to maintain and continue the effect.
4. Many patients will eventually require surgical resection of the infiltrated lip. After surgery intralesional triamcinolone acetonide may be used to treat or prevent recurrence.

Pitfalls

1. Repeated triamcinolone injections in the lip may lead to atrophy or weakness.
2. Cheilitis *glandularis* may closely mimic cheilitis *granulomatosa*. A biopsy will help to differentiate, as will squeezing the lip and demonstrating the hyperplastic salivary glands in the former.

TB

27

Chloasma

Facial Melanosis, Melasma

Facial melanosis usually appears in association with OCP use or pregnancy ("chloasma," or the "mask of pregnancy"), and is exacerbated by sun exposure. Although the pigmentation usually fades after pregnancy or withdrawal of OCPs, it may persist indefinitely.

Initial Therapy

1. Patients whose pigmentation is enhanced when examined under Wood's light are more likely to respond to therapy.
2. To eliminate pre-existing pigmentation, apply hydroquinone 4% cream b.i.d. *only* to hyperpigmented areas for 6 weeks.

Alternate Therapy

1. Retinoic acid (Retin-A) 0.05% cream q.h.s. is almost as effective as hydroquinone for eliminating hyperpigmentation.

Subsequent Therapy

1. If no depigmentation has occurred after 6 weeks of therapy with hydroquinone alone, add retinoic acid 0.05% cream q.h.s., or utilize a 1 : 1 mixture

of hydroquinone 4% and retinoic acid 0.1% (irritation from retinoic acid can be controlled by concurrent application of low-potency topical steroid (e.g., desonide or hydrocortisone 2.5% cream)).
2. Advise the patient to minimize exposure to sunlight and other UV sources.
3. Daily application of a sunscreen with a UVA blocking ingredient (benzophenone or cinnamate), preferably SPF 15 or higher.

Pitfalls

1. Hydroquinone also will lighten normal skin; hence, care should be taken to apply it only to affected areas.
2. Even after satisfactory treatment melanosis will recur if sun exposure is not kept to a minimum; hence, sunscreens should be employed indefinitely.
3. Both hydroquinone and retinoic acid can be irritating and even sensitizing. Inclusion of a low-potency topical steroid can minimize the irritancy, but not the possibility of sensitization.

PE

28

Chondrodermatitis Nodularis Helicis

Initial Therapy

1. Intralesional triamcinolone acetonide 5 mg/cc is injected into the dermis and perichondrium of the affected area.
2. Advise the patient to avoid all pressure to the area. Recommend using a soft pillow or "doughnut," holding the telephone receiver against the other ear, and avoiding headphones.

Alternative Therapy

1. Cryotherapy, as for a hypertrophic actinic keratosis.
2. Although expensive, injection of a tiny bit of bovine collagen (Zyderm)

under the tender area will occasionally lead to healing. (First perform a skin test to rule out allergy to bovine collagen.)

Subsequent Therapy

Most areas are recurrent and relapsing, and eventually require surgical excision of the affected area *and* a small portion of subjacent cartilage.

Pitfalls

1. A small actinic keratosis or squamous cell carcinoma may clinically resemble chondrodermatitis nodularis helicis. If there is any doubt a biopsy is warranted.
2. Inadequate depth and extent of surgery may lead to recurrence.

TB

29

Chronic Bullous Disease of Childhood

Chronic bullous disease of childhood is characterized by the presence of multiple, tense bullae and severe itching in association with linear deposition of IgA at the basement membrane zone. The clinical appearance resembles bullous pemphigoid. It often remits 2–3 years after onset, and rarely lasts past age 10.

Initial Therapy

1. Treat with either dapsone 2 mg/kg/day or sulfapyridine 35–70 mg/kg/day.
2. If no improvement is noted after 5 days, increase the dosage of either drug at 5-day intervals until an efficacious dose is reached. Sulfapyridine 200 mg–3 g/day or dapsone 25–125 mg/day may be required. Either drug may be crushed in a flavored syrup. Monitor CBC prior to each increase in sulfone dose.

Subsequent Therapy

When the disease is controlled, taper either drug to the dose required to maintain patient comfort. Attempt to wean the patient off medication at 4- or 6-month intervals. Recheck the CBC every 2 months while the patient is receiving maintenance sulfones.

Alternative Therapy

1. Although most children respond to sulfones, addition of corticosteroids (e.g., prednisone) may be required to achieve control.
2. If control is not possible with 3 g of sulfapyridine or 125 mg of dapsone, add prednisone 1 mg/kg/day and attempt to convert to a q.o.d. steroid schedule as quickly as possible.

Pitfalls

1. Because this is a benign, self-limited disorder, patient comfort rather than total suppression of disease activity is the therapeutic goal. Accept limited disease activity and do not overtreat with steroids or sulfones in relatively recalcitrant cases.
2. Screen all patients for G6PD activity prior to beginning sulfone therapy.

BW

30

Cicatricial Pemphigoid

Cicatricial pemphigoid is a chronic, scarring bullous disorder that affects mucous membranes, including the conjunctivae. The therapeutic goal is to prevent blindness caused by conjunctival scarring and to control the symptoms or the nutritional problems caused by mucous membrane lesions. Unfortunately, cicatricial pemphigoid is difficult to treat, and blindness may not always be avoided.

Initial Therapy

1. Dapsone 100 mg/day may be used in patients without conjunctival involvement or with little inflammatory mucous membrane involvement. If improvement is not noted after 2 weeks, increase dose by 100 mg/day every 2 weeks until control is achieved. Do not exceed 400 mg/day. This drug may also be used in combination with prednisone 60–80 mg/day.
2. For severe disease or disease with conjunctival involvement, treat with prednisone 60–80 mg/day in combination with azathioprine (Imuran) 100–200 mg/day. When disease control is achieved, taper the prednisone to a q.o.d. schedule and maintain azathioprine at the lowest dose necessary for control.

Alternative Therapy

Cyclophosphamide 100–200 mg/day in combination with prednisone has been used, but is not clearly superior to azathioprine. Cyclophosphamide side effects of hemorrhagic cystitis and leukemia make this a less attractive regimen.

Adjunctive Therapy

1. Frequently applied (t.i.d. or q.i.d.) high-potency topical steroids may be used for skin or mucous membrane lesions.
2. Symptoms of oral ulcerations may require, as necessary, use of topical anesthetics such as viscous lidocaine 2% washes.

Pitfalls

1. Do not forget ophthalmic consultation. Blindness is the most-feared complication of this disorder, occurring in 25%–50% of cases. Joint management is essential to assess and document conjunctival involvement in all phases of diagnosis and therapy.
2. In dapsone-treated patients, monitor CBC every 2 weeks while the dose is raised, and every 3–6 weeks after a maintenance dose is established.

BW

31

Coccidioidomycosis (and Paracoccidioidomycosis)

For practical purposes, coccidioidomycosis occurs only in residents or visitors to the Southwestern United States. Blacks (14-fold increase) and Filipinos (175-fold increase) have a much higher rate of dissemination than Caucasians. Paracoccidioidomycosis occurs primarily in Caucasians (10 times more often in males than in females), and only in inhabitants of South and Central America. In the majority of infected individuals (those having the localized form), illness is mild and heals spontaneously; however, the disseminated form is serious and must be treated as early as possible. In coccidioidomycosis, dissemination is far more likely to occur in Filipinos and blacks and in the immunosuppressed.

Initial Therapy

Intravenous amphotericin B (Fungizone) is standard therapy. The dose is 25 mg, diluted in 150 ml of 5% glucose in water (containing hydrocortisone 25–50 mg and heparin 250–1,000 U), administered over 24 hours. The usual dose is 20–30 mg/day for a total of 4–6 weeks, with the total dose not to exceed 3 g. To reduce acute reactions, premedicate patients with diphenhydramine (Benadryl) 50–100 mg plus meperidine (Demerol) 25–100 mg, 15 minutes prior to infusions. Note: For patients with meningeal involvement, amphotericin must be given intrathecally as well.

Alternative Therapy

1. Imidazole antifungal agents are not as effective as amphotericin (only 35% cure and high relapse rate). Oral ketoconazole (Nizoral) 400–1,200 mg/day or intravenous micronozole (Micatin) 25 mg/kg/day, in either saline or glucose, divided into three daily infusions, can be administered alone to those patients who do not tolerate amphotericin or those with mild disease. Ketoconazole therapy sometimes must be given for 6–18 months before the

patient is completely disease free. Amphotericin B can be administered along with one of these agents to patients with severe, refractory, or disseminated disease.

2. Transfer factor reportedly has benefitted some patients with disseminated or refractory disease.
3. Sulfonamides are reportedly suppressive for mild cases of paracoccidioidomycosis.

Ancillary Therapy

1. Surgical drainage and/or debridement may be required for encapsulated abscesses or avascular necrotic lesions.
2. Ventriculovascular, -peritoneal, or -pleural shunts may be required in patients with meningeal disease, who develop persistent elevations of CSF pressure.

Pitfalls

1. Relapses of coccidioidomycosis are common, especially in patients treated with imidazole agents.
2. Pregnancy is an adverse risk factor in coccidioidomycosis: dissemination is far more common.
3. Disseminated coccidioidomycosis results from hematogenous spread of the fungus. Subcutaneous abscesses, cellulitis, and draining sinuses are the cutaneous hallmarks, although bone and meninges are frequently involved. A negative skin test to coccidioidin with rising antibody titers suggests impending dissemination.
4. As with all systemic mycoses, erythema nodosum can occur.
5. Amphotericin B can produce cardiac toxicity if infused too rapidly. Reactions, including chills, fever, nausea, malaise, and anorexia, although reversible, can be severe. These symptoms can be aborted by preadministration of diphenhydramine and meperidine, as well as coadministration of hydrocortisone intravenously with drug infusions (see below). Salicylates and antihistamines are less effective, but occasionally useful. Kidney function must be monitored closely (e.g., twice-weekly BUN and creatinine) and therapy should be interrupted for at least 1 day whenever creatinine levels exceed 3 mg%. Heparin (1000 U/infusion) should be included in the infusions to minimize the risk of phlebitis. Other side effects that should be looked for include hypokalemia, hypomagnesemia, and anemia.
6. Side effects of ketoconazole rarely can include severe hepatoxicity (monitor with pretreatment and serial liver enzyme measurements, i.e., every 3–4 weeks), gynecomastia, impotence, and oligospermia. The last three are

due to inhibition of adrenal or gonadal steroid and/or testosterone synthesis. Usually normal hormone function resumes by 3 weeks after discontinuation of the drug.

PE

32

Cold Injury: Chilblains

Pernio

Chilblains represent an abnormal reaction to cold that occurs primarily in women, children, and the elderly. Lesions tend to become worse in the elderly, and improve spontaneously in younger patients.

Initial Therapy

The calcium channel blockers nifedipine (Procardia) 10 mg t.i.d. and diltiazam (Cardizem) 30 mg t.i.d. usually will prevent recurrent episodes of chilblains. Monitor blood pressure at the start of treatment and at return visits.

Ancillary Therapy

1. Warm clothing and a warm climate are usually more helpful than drugs. Abrupt changes in temperature are particularly harmful, and should be avoided.
2. Weight reduction and exercise are helpful in reducing susceptibility to recurrent episodes of chilblains.
3. Keep feet dry. Moisture enhances cold injury.

Alternative Therapy

1. Nicotinamide 500 mg t.i.d. may be useful alone or in addition to calcium channel blockers. Increase the dose as tolerated to 1 g t.i.d.

2. Phenoxybenzamine (Dibenzyline) 10 mg/day increasing to b.i.d. can be tried in cases unresponsive to nicotinamide.
3. Erythematous doses of ultraviolet light (UVB) to affected areas 2–3 ×/week at the start of winter may help.
4. Sympathectomy is sometimes required for severe, unremitting cases.

Pitfalls

1. Pernio-like lesions occur in both discoid and systemic lupus erythematosus, as well as in sarcoidosis. The possibility of lupus should be excluded by appropriate laboratory tests (see Ch. 169) and biopsy.
2. Chilblains may be accompanied by other clinical manifestations of cold sensitivity, such as acrocyanosis and/or erythrocyanosis.

PE

33

Cold Injury: Frostbite

Acute frostbite (less than 24 hours following exposure) is a relative medical emergency, requiring measures different from those for chronic frostbite injury.

Initial Therapy

1. For acute frostbite only: Immediately immerse the exposed body part in warm water (104–108°F) for 15–30 minutes. Do not attempt rewarming until the victim is in an appropriate treatment facility.
2. Administer phenoxybenzamine (Dibenzyline) 10 mg/day for 10 days.
3. Administer acetylsalicylic acid (aspirin) 5 g q6h to reduce platelet aggregation.
4. Administer Penicillin VK 250 mg q.6h. until the edema resolves to reduce possibility of secondary (usually streptococcal) infection.

Ancillary Therapy

1. Elevate, splint, and protect (using a cradle for feet and cotton between digits) the affected parts.
2. Administer tetanus toxoid if indicated.
3. Administer an analgesic, morphine, meperidine plus promethazine, or propoxyphene napsylate, depending on severity of pain.
4. An anxiolytic (e.g., diazepam) and/or sleeping medication (e.g., tenazepam) may be needed.
5. A high-calorie, high-protein diet is indicated.
6. Encourage the patient to stop smoking and desist from any other nicotine intake.
7. Encourage constant digital exercise for fingers and toes to help reestablish circulation.
8. A whirlpool bath with povidone-iodine (Betadine) b.i.d. is useful for debridement and to prevent secondary infections.

Pitfalls

1. Deep frostbite injury can cause bone changes, and in children epiphyseal necrosis can result in digital deformation.
2. Because prolonged freezing is less injurious than repeated freeze-thawing, warming should not be undertaken until the patient reaches a treatment facility if the possibility of refreezing exists.

PE

34

Contact Dermatitis

Contact dermatitis can have either an irritant or an allergic origin. Irritant reactions tend to appear less than 12 hours after exposure, and are strictly limited to exposed sites. Allergic reactions are delayed (12–72 hours, except for primary sensitization, where an induction phase of 7–10 days is typical), and exhibit a tendency to spread as the delayed hypersensitivity reaction reaches sites where less antigen was deposited initially.

Initial Therapy

LIMITED AREAS OF INVOLVEMENT

1. Treat with cool compresses, using Domeboro tablets or packets, one tablet or packet in 1 pt of tap water. A clean washcloth or towel should be used and applied wet (but not soaking wet) to the rash for 15–20 minutes b.i.d.
2. Prescribe a potent topical fluorinated steroid preparation in a drying vehicle (e.g., fluocinonide gel) to be applied b.i.d. to the rash. *Note:* For acute contact dermatitis on the face or intertriginous areas, a nonfluorinated, nonatrophogenic topical steroid (e.g., desonide (Tridesilon) or hydrocortisone 2.5% cream (Hytone) is preferable.
3. For additional relief of pruritus an astringent lotion, with or without additional ingredients such as menthol, camphor, and phenol in low concentration (≤1%) (e.g., Sarna), can be applied as frequently as needed.
4. If pruritus is interfering with sleep, low doses of antihistamines (e.g., chlorpheniramine, 4–8 mg q.h.s.) can be prescribed, and a nonsoporiphic antihistamine (e.g., clemastine (Tavist) 1 tablet b.i.d. or terfenadine (Seldane) 60 mg b.i.d.) can be administered if relief is needed during waking hours.

WIDESPREAD INVOLVEMENT

1. Systemic steroids: Topical steroids are only minimally effective for acute contact dermatitis. Therefore, as disease becomes more generalized and/or involves face, genitalia, or other areas that compromise normal activity, a course of systemic steroids may be indicated. For re-exposure (as in recurrent episodes of poison ivy or poison oak), a 10–14-day tapering course of prednisone, beginning with 50 or 60 mg/day, is indicated. Administer each day's medication as a single morning dose taken with food or a glass of milk to reduce the likelihood of stomach upset.

   For patients with *primary sensitization*, where the course may extend up to 4–6 weeks, a single intramuscular injection of triamcinolone acetonide 40–60 mg total, together with an additional 1 cc of betamethasone valerate (Celestone), will provide a fairly rapid onset of action and prolonged action over 2–4 weeks. *Note:* Intramuscular steroids should be administered deeply intramuscularly in the buttocks to avoid possible atrophy of overlying subcutaneous fat.

   As a further precaution, in all patients who are candidates for systemic steroids, ascertain the presence or absence of absolute or relative contraindications to steroid therapy (e.g., cases of active peptic ulcer disease, diabetes, hypertension, psychiatric disease, tuberculosis, HIV infection, and abnormal menses. Note: Women should be warned that these doses of steroids can cause short-term irregularities or decreased menses).

2. Cool baths with oilated colloidal oatmeal (Aveeno) can provide substantial, temporary relief for patients with extensive disease.
3. Secondary bacterial infection, although uncommon, may occur, and can be hard to detect in extensive contact dermatitis. Administer oral systemic antibiotics, such as erythromycin or dicloxacillin 1 g/day to patients with obvious infections. Early or suspected infections can be treated with antibacterial cleansers (e.g., chlorhexidine (Hibiclens) or povidone iodine (Betadine)) and/or topical antibiotics (e.g., bacitracin, triple antibiotic cream, or mupirocin (Bactroban)).

Subsequent Therapy

Search for the suspected irritant/allergen: In most cases of contact dermatitis, the cause is apparent, but some cases may require patch testing to pinpoint the culprit (e.g., in shoes, clothing, and deodorants many potential contactants are present together). Patch tests are best performed by physicians experienced in these procedures.

Pitfalls

1. The pitfalls of both topical and systemic steroid therapy are discussed in Appendices 4 and 5.
2. The possibility of secondary infection is discussed above.
3. Irritant reactions are often confused with allergic dermatitis by both patients and physicians. Yet the distinction is important because irritant reactions are concentration dependent. Therefore, certain agents that are irritants in one bodily site may be safe to use in another site (e.g., aluminum chloride may be an irritant in occluded, intertriginous areas but nonreactive when used as an astringent on the palms, soles, or back).
4. Airborne contact dermatitis can be difficult to distinguish from photoallergy or phototoxicity. An important clue is extension of the rash to the neck, submental, and/or infranasal areas.

PE

35

Creeping Eruption

There are two forms of creeping eruption: larva migrans, usually due to an animal or rarely a human hookworm, and larva currens, caused by *S. stercoralis*. Larva migrans is usually self-limited, whereas larva currens is usually chronic.

Initial Therapy

For larva migrans only thiabendazole 10% suspension may be applied to the lesions t.i.d. to q.i.d.

Alternative Therapy

For larva migrans and larva currens, oral thiabendazole 25 mg/kg b.i.d. for 2–3 days is usually adequate to control the infestation.

Pitfall

Numerous adverse reactions have been reported with oral thiabendazole. Physicians prescribing this medication should be alert for potential drug reactions.

TB

36

Cutaneous Candidiasis

C. albicans causes cutaneous disease in occluded, moist areas: the groin, axilla, inframammary areas, and the glans penis (in uncircumcised males). Diabetes, obesity, fecal and urinary incontinence, and immunosuppression are predisposing factors.

Initial Therapy

1. If the skin is weeping, instruct the patient to soak in dilute Burow's solution 1 : 40 b.i.d. for 15 minutes.
2. Prescribe nystatin ointment applied t.i.d. or an imidazole cream applied b.i.d. to the affected area. If erosive lesions are present the cream may cause burning.
3. Instruct the patient to dry the moist areas by exposing them to the air, and to keep stool and urine away from the skin.
4. Look for associated yeast vaginitis in cases of vulvar candidiasis in women.
5. Suspect GI tract overgrowth in cases of perianal candidiasis. Add oral nystatin 500,000 U t.i.d. for 1 week.
6. Evaluate the patient for diabetes mellitus.

Subsequent Therapy

1. Nystatin ointment or zinc oxide paste applied over the topical imidazole may enhance therapy by providing a protective barrier from sweat, urine, and stool.
2. Adding hydrocortisone 1% ointment to the anticandidal agent will speed healing and reduce symptoms more rapidly.
3. Men with balanitis often have partners with candidal vaginitis; they also need treatment. In refractory cases circumcision may help, but is rarely necessary.
4. Although cosmetically unattractive, gentian violet solution b.i.d. × 3 days is drying and has good anticandidal activity.
5. For severe unresponsive cases oral ketoconazole 200 mg/day for 1–2 weeks is of benefit.
6. Preventive therapy includes keeping the area dry by wearing loose-fitting underwear and using topical drying powders (e.g., Zeasorb).

Pitfalls

1. Do a KOH preparation prior to therapy to establish the diagnosis.
2. Secondary bacterial infection may require systemic antibiotics.
3. Avoid applying solutions to inflamed skin, as they will cause burning.
4. Refractory lesions may need a biopsy to rule out extramammary Paget's disease, squamous cell carcinoma in situ (Bowen's disease), and metabolic and other inflammatory causes of an intertriginous eruption.
5. Oral ketoconazole may cause liver function abnormalities.

PE

37

Cutaneous Cysts

Four types of cutaneous cysts are discussed; epidermal inclusion cysts (mistakenly called sebaceous cysts), pilar cysts (wens), digital mucinous or ganglion cysts, and median raphe cysts or sinus of the penis. Patients with pilonidal cysts should be referred to a general surgeon for treatment.

EPIDERMAL INCLUSION CYSTS AND PILAR CYSTS

Initial Therapy

UNINFLAMED CYST

If the cyst is uninflamed surgical therapy is optimal.

1. Complete surgical excision with primary closure gives good results and the recurrence rate is very low.
2. Alternatively, after local anesthesia the cyst may be lanced with a #11 blade, the contents expressed, and the wall curetted out. Although cysts may recur following this therapy, it is a good alternative as initial treatment in a cosmetically sensitive area for cysts under 7 mm. If they don't recur almost no scar results. This technique is especially good for pilar cysts of any size. Curettage and suturing are often not required after expressing pilar cysts.

INFLAMED CYST

Do not excise an inflamed cyst as its margins cannot be determined and operative bleeding is significant.

1. Intralesional triamcinolone acetonide 2.5–5 mg/cc may be injected in and around the inflamed cyst to reduce erythema and pain.
2. If the inflamed cyst is fluctuant, perform incision and drainage. If the contents are purulent, perform a bacterial culture. A Gram stain is indicated if suspicion of infection is high. Use a curette to remove all the

keratinous debris, and irrigate the wound to wash out any loose fragments. Careful removal of the cyst wall in pieces with pickups and fine scissors may reduce the need for a follow-up excision. If a large defect results pack it with gauze for a few days. Cleanse the resulting defect with hydrogen peroxide b.i.d. once the packing is removed until it is healed.

Subsequent Therapy

1. Surgically excise recurrent cysts with wider margins.
2. Once inflamed cysts are no longer erythematous or if they recur after incision and drainage, they may be surgically excised. Wait at least one month after initial treatment before surgical excision.

Pitfalls

1. Inflamed cysts and bacterial abscesses often cannot be differentiated. Incision and drainage is indicated if the cyst is fluctuant. A Gram stain of the contents may help in this differential diagnosis.
2. Inflamed cysts usually result from rupture of the cyst wall and an intense foreign-body reaction, not from infection. Oral antibiotics are only indicated if other signs of infection are present or if a Gram stain or culture of the purulent material reveals a pathogen.
3. Always send excised cysts for pathologic examination.

DIGITAL MUCINOUS AND GANGLION CYSTS

Initial Therapy

1. Cysts may be drained by incising with a #11 blade or a large needle and expressing the gelatinous contents. Repeated drainage alone may lead to resolution.
2. Triamcinolone acetonide 5 mg/cc may be injected in the cyst and the surrounding tissue after it has been incised and drained.

Subsequent

1. Splinting of an affected digit for several weeks after draining the cyst may reduce recurrence. The possibility of a frozen joint must be avoided.
2. Liquid nitrogen cryotherapy with freeze times of 30 seconds may be effective for digital cysts.

3. Surgical excision of the digital cyst and the surrounding proximal nail fold has a low recurrence rate. The resultant surgical defect requires 6–10 weeks to heal. Infection of the surgical wound may damage the superficial extensor tendon. This surgery should only be performed on healthy, compliant patients by physicians experienced in surgery.
4. Refer patients with ganglions of the wirst recurring after drainage and intralesional steroid therapy to an orthopaedic or hand surgeon.

Pitfalls

1. Inform the patient before any treatment is given that recurrence is common.
2. Infection of cysts near joints can be serious. Use careful sterile technique for even the simplest procedure.
3. Triamcinolone injected into tissue may be carried proximally along lymphatics, creating narrow bands of atrophy, hypopigmentation, and alopecia. Inform the patient of this potential complication.

MEDIAN RAPHE CYSTS AND SINUSES

Initial Therapy

Surgical excision is usually curative.

Pitfalls

These cysts may occasionally connect to the urethra. If the cyst or sinus does not dissect out cleanly, consult a urologist.

TB

38

Cutaneous Horn

Cutaneous horn is a clinical term for a hyperkeratotic lesion whose keratinous cap is sufficient to protrude from the skin. It may overlie a benign or malignant lesion.

Initial Therapy

1. In young patients and in those without significant sun damage, the lesion can usually be frozen, as it is almost always benign. Pigmented lesions are an exception and should be biopsied.
2. Biopsy a cutaneous horn in older persons, and in those with significant sun damage. If the lesion appears to have a dermal component a complete excision will provide an optimum specimen for diagnosis, and is also usually curative.

Subsequent Therapy

Biopsy any cutaneous horn not responding to cryotherapy.

Pitfalls

1. Failure to biopsy a malignant lesion may delay the diagnosis.
2. A shave biopsy of cutaneous horn often does not include the base of the lesion. This prevents adequate pathologic interpretation. A "scoop" or deep shave, or preferably a small ellipse, is recommended.

TB

39

Cutaneous T-Cell Lymphoma

Mycosis Fungoides • Sézary Syndrome

Therapy of cutaneous T-cell lymphoma has not been standardized, and often requires specialized knowledge. For this reason, it is often appropriate to refer such patients for consultation. The most useful of the many therapeutic modalities available for treatment of this complex disease will be described in detail. Appropriate alternatives for each stage of the disease are listed at the end of this section. Since no therapy is known to cure this disorder, the therapeutic goal is always to control the process and reduce cutaneous lesions in an effort to maintain a high quality of life.

THERAPEUTIC MODALITIES

Topical Therapy

1. Topical nitrogen mustard: A solution of nitrogen mustard 10 mg dissolved in 50–60 ml of tap water is applied q.d. to the entire skin, except the scalp, eyelids, axillae, and perineum, using a nylon paint brush until clearing is achieved (the perineum may be painted with a 1 : 1 solution). Unused material may be stored in the refrigerator for at least a week. After the solution dries, the skin is covered with an emollient (e.g., Eucerin, Aquaphor). Some advocate q.d. (or q.o.d.) application for months or even years to maintain remission. Approximately 30% of patients will be sensitized by this regimen.

2. Topical carmustine (BCNU): Topical carmustine may be applied to the entire body or to localized skin lesions.

   a. Therapy of localized lesions: Carmustine is supplied in 20-mg vials; 10 ml of 95% alcohol is added to each, dissolved, and saved as 0.2% Carmustine stock solution. A cotton-tipped applicator is used to apply the stock solution directly to each lesion b.i.d. for 2 weeks; therapy may be repeated after a 6-week rest period. Monitor CBC and platelets weekly during treatment. If lesions become noticeably irritated, application of carmustine is ceased and instead a fluorinated topical steroid is applied q.i.d.

   b. Whole-body therapy: A solution of 10 ml of the carmustine 0.2% stock solution and 60 ml (2 oz) of cool tap water is mixed in a clearly labelled glass container (not a paper cup). After a lukewarm shower, the entire solution is applied to the body, including the face, scalp, palms and soles, but sparing genitals, groins, armpits, bends or elbows, behind knees and inframammary folds, unless these have active lesions, using a 2-inch nylon paint brush. The total body may be treated q.d. for 14 days. Obtain a CBC and a platelet count initially and every 2 weeks during treatment. The patient may be retreated after an 8-week rest period; resistant plaques can be treated using the protocol for therapy of localized lesions (above).

   c. Side effects include erythema, irritant dermatitis, urticaria, telangiectasia, and reversible bone marrow depression with pancytopenia.

Systemic Therapy

1. Photochemotherapy (PUVA): Administer psoralen 0.6 mg/kg 2 hours before UVA exposure. Treat 3 ×/week until lesions clear, and then taper therapy with the goal of treating the patient once every 3–4 weeks. Select initial UVA exposure on the basis of skin type.
   a. For patients who always sunburn and never tan, start with 1.5–3.0 J/m^2;
   b. For patients who always sunburn and sometimes tan, start with 2.5–5.0 J/m^2;
   c. For patients who sometimes sunburn but always tan, start with 3.5–7.0 J/m^2;
   d. For patients who never sunburn and always tan, start with 4.5–9.0 J/m^2;
   e. For patients who are moderately pigmented, start with 5.5–11.0 J/m^2;
   f. For blacks, start with 6.5–13.0 J/m^2.
   Increase UVA exposure by 0.5 J/m^2 each treatment. The patient must wear UVA-filtering eyeglasses the entire day of therapy, and should be examined by an ophthalmologist at initiation of treatment and every 6 months during treatment. Early side effects include nausea following psoralen administration, phototoxic erythema, pruritus, and variable pigmentation. Late side effects include skin carcinogenesis, enhanced photoaging, pigmentary changes, and ocular damage.
2. Chemotherapy
   a. Methotrexate, when not contraindicated, may be used as the sole chemotherapeutic agent. Contraindications include decreased renal function, significantly abnormal liver function, recent or active hepatitis, cirrhosis, excessive alcohol consumption, severe leukopenia, thrombocytopenia, anemia, active peptic ulcer, active severe infectious diseases, and an unreliable patient.
      Begin with a single test dose of oral or intravenous methotrexate 5 mg/week. Increase the dose by 5–10 mg/week, if tolerated, until 50 mg is reached. Monitor CBC and platelet count weekly while increasing dosage, and at monthly intervals when the dose is stabilized. If side effects such as oral ulceration, GI upset, suppression of CBC and platelet count, or alteration of LFTs are encountered, discontinue therapy; following the patient's recovery from a side effect, attempt to achieve the methotrexate dosage just below that associated with toxicity. Obtain a liver biopsy initially and after 1.5-gm therapy.
   b. Combined-agent chemotherapy may be attempted, although it is not described here in detail. These agents may include cyclophos-

phamide, vincristine, and prednisone with or without bleomycin; cyclophosphamide, doxorubicin, vincristine, and prednisone; and chlorambucil and prednisone.

3. Photopheresis: This is a form of photochemotherapy using extracorporeal irradiation of peripheral blood leukocytes that have been photosensitized with psoralen at a dose of 0.6 mg/ml. Two hours later, using a photopheresis device, the peripheral blood leukocytes are harvested, exposed to UVA light, and then reinfused into the patient. The procedure is carried out in specialized centers and requires treatments on 2 consecutive days every fifth week for 6–12 treatments to induce a successful clinical response.

Electron Beam Therapy

Whole-body electron beam therapy is given by radiation oncology specialists. The electron beam treats the entire skin to a controlled depth of 1–2 cm. The optimal total dosage is 3,000–3,600 rads given over an 8–9-week period in 200-rad fractions. Localized lesions may be treated with spot therapy using 600–1,200 rads.

Pitfalls

Side effects include erythroderma and desquamation, with or without edema and blistering, hyperpigmentation, reversible hair loss, onycholysis, epidermal atrophy, telangiectasia, actinic keratosis, keratoacanthoma, and basal or squamous cell carcinoma. Each patient may be treated only once, and for this reason, electron beam therapy should be used only in patients who do not respond to more benign forms of therapy.

THERAPY OF CUTANEOUS T-CELL LYMPHOMA

Therapeutic approaches to cutaneous T-cell lymphoma differ depending on the clinical stage of the disease and the practice of the therapist. Thus, the many therapeutic options are presented as unranked alternatives for each clinical stage.

Stage IA

Premycotic lesions, papules, or plaques involving *less* than 10% of the skin, *without* lymph node involvement.

1. Local nitrogen mustard.
2. Local carmustine.
3. PUVA.

Stage IB

Premycotic lesions, papules, or plaques involving *more* than 10% of the skin, *without* lymph node involvement.

1. Whole-body nitrogen mustard.
2. Whole-body carmustine.
3. PUVA.
4. Photopheresis with or without methotrexate.
5. Methotrexate.
6. Electron beam therapy.

Stage IIA

Premycotic lesions, papules, or plaques involving *more* than 10% of the skin, *with* clinical lymph node involvement.

1. Whole-body nitrogen mustard.
2. Whole-body carmustine.
3. PUVA.
4. Photopheresis with or without methotrexate.
5. Methotrexate.
6. Electron beam therapy.

Stage IIB

Skin tumors with or without clinical lymph node involvement.

1. Electron beam therapy.
2. Methotrexate.
3. Combined-agent chemotherapy.
4. Photopheresis with methotrexate.

Stage III

Generalized erythroderma with or without clinical lymph node involvement.

1. Nitrogen mustard.
2. Photopheresis with or without methotrexate.
3. Methotrexate.
4. Combined-agent chemotherapy.
5. Electron beam therapy.
6. Electron beam therapy with combined-agent chemotherapy.

Stages IVA and B

Patches, plaques, tumors or erythroderma with pathologically involved nodes.

1. Electron beam therapy with combined-agent chemotherapy.
2. Appropriate experimental regimens.

BW

40

Darier's Disease

Keratosis Follicularis

The diagnosis of Darier's disease is dependent on clinical features: family history and a characteristic histopathology. Two clinical patterns can be distinguished: a "seborrheic" form of the disease, with clinical similarities to Hailey–Hailey disease, and a cornifying variant, characterized by hypertrophic, vegetative lesions, primarily on the lower extremities. Because of seasonal exacerbations and partial remissions, therapy should be adjusted accordingly.

Initial Therapy

1. The currently accepted primary treatment of moderate-to-severe Darier's disease is with systemic retinoids (isotretinoin, etretinate, and acitretin are equally effective, but higher doses of isotretinoin (with a greater incidence of toxicity) may be required to achieve an equivalent result). Etretinate 1–

2 mg/kg/day or acitretin 0.5–1 mg/kg/day should be given in divided doses (the initial dose is dictated by disease severity). *Note:* Because of possible long-term musculoskeletal toxicity (see below), do not administer retinoids to growing children. Retinoids should be administered only by physicians who possess expertise with these drugs.

2. For mild or localized disease topical retinoic acid 0.025% gel or 0.1% cream q.h.s. may suffice for patients with mild or limited disease.

Ancillary and Subsequent Therapy

1. As soon as a good response to systemic retinoids is observed (i.e., usually after about 4–8 weeks), reduce the daily retinoid dose quickly. Maintenance therapy constitutes the lowest dose that suppresses the most severe disease features; q.o.d. regimens can be employed in an attempt to further reduce long-term toxicity (however, the efficacy of this approach in reducing toxicity is still unproven). Finally, since the disease tends to be relatively quiescent during winter months, if possible, discontinue retinoid therapy completely for several months, thereby potentially minimizing long-term side effects.

2. Flares of Darier's disease are often precipitated by secondary infections owing both to a defective skin barrier and to minor immunologic dysfunction in this disease. Hence, therapy often includes an initial 10–14-day course of a bacteriocidal antibiotic (e.g., oral dicloxacillin 250 mg q.i.d.) aimed at coagulase-positive *S. aureus*, the most commonly encountered pathogen. In penicillin-allergic individuals, trimethoprim-sulfamethoxazole (Bactrim DS or Septra DS) 1 tablet b.i.d., cephalexin 250 mg q.i.d., or ciprofloxacin 500 mg t.i.d. may be employed. Obtain cultures and sensitivities routinely, as patients with Darier's disease often develop antibiotic-resistant pathogens following frequent courses of antibiotic therapy (see Pitfalls).

3. Because Darier's disease often appears to flare after acute exposure to sunlight (UVB is the active wavelength), instruct patients to apply a PABA–benzophenone-containing sunscreen (SPF 15 or higher) daily from March to October, and year-round in more Southern latitudes.

4. Heat, sweating, and friction can exacerbate Darier's disease, either directly or indirectly via secondary bacterial infections. Hence, patients should bathe with an antibacterial cleanser, such as povidone iodine (Betadine) or chlorhexidine (Hibiclens), daily. Additional helpful measures include application of aluminum chloride 6% suspension (Xerac AC) q.d. to intertriginous, disease-prone areas, followed by application of an astringent powder, such as Zeasorb.

5. Patients with a history of frequent bacterial superinfections may benefit

from prophylactic topical antibiotics, such as clindamycin 1% (Cleocin T) solution or erythromycin 2% q.d. to disease-prone areas.

Pitfalls

1. Some patients with the seborrheic variant of keratosis follicularis may be worsened by systemic retinoids owing to the tendency of these agents to cause epidermal fragility. However, failure with one retinoid does not necessarily preclude the use of others. Thus, etretinate-resistant cases may benefit from isotretinoin and vice-versa. If both retinoids cause worsening of disease, the patient must be managed with the other conservative measures described above.
2. Frequent courses of oral antibiotics often result in colonization by semi-synthetic penicillin- or cephalosporin-resistant strains of staphylococci.
3. As described above, secondary infections owing to heat and excessive friction, as well as to acute exposure to ultraviolet light, can cause disease flares.
4. Systemic retinoids can cause both acute and chronic side effects (see Appendix 6). Hence, patients must be fully aware of the risks and benefits of this therapy.

PE

41

Decubitus Ulcer

Initial Therapy

The therapeutic goal is to encourage formation of healthy granulation tissue and a clean ulcer base.

1. General measures
   a. Maintain adequate nutrition.
   b. Maintain movement by any measures necessary in order to ensure that the lesion is not compressed and that bony prominences are not immobilized. A Clinitron air bed or a soft mattress may be required.

2. Debride the ulcer to allow formation of granulation tissue; apply wet-to-dry dressings t.i.d. or debride the ulcer surgically.
3. Send the ulcer contents for culture and sensitivity; treat with an appropriate antibiotic if a pathogen is present.

Subsequent Therapy

When the ulcer is clean and healthy granulation tissue is present:

1. Fill the ulcer with Duoderm beads and cover it with a Duoderm occlusive dressing; change the dressing weekly or sooner if the Duoderm becomes too "soupy."
2. Complete healing may take months. BE PATIENT.
3. If not significantly improved after 2–3 months, consider a skin graft.

Pitfalls

1. Inadequate nutrition will prevent healing regardless of the therapy employed.
2. Of the many therapeutic agents formerly employed in ulcer care, including benzoyl peroxide, milk, diphenhydramine (Benadryl), topical antibiotics, and many others, none is necessary if the physician is patient and the care meticulous; a complicating contact dermatitis can thus be avoided.
3. Improper diagnosis. Cutaneous carcinoma (basal cell, squamous cell) may cause ulceration that may be confused with decubiti.

BW

42

Delusions of Parasitosis

The patient with delusions of parasitosis holds a fixed belief of infestation by ectoparasites despite clinical evidence to the contrary; logic and reassurance are ineffective. The condition is often associated with folie à deux, in which the patient's intimate associate(s) share and reinforce the patient's belief system. The diagnosis is confirmed by eliminating other possibilities. Confronting the patient with a direct statement of a psychogenic nature of the diagnosis should be avoided until an adequate rapport is established, otherwise subsequent treatment will be more difficult or impossible.

Initial Therapy

1. Concentrate therapy on relief of symptoms. Although the patient may disagree with the diagnosis, relief of symptoms (or the desire for such relief) helps build the trust necessary for subsequent rapport and willingness to participate in definitive therapy.
2. Treatment is with the antipsychotic pimozide (Orap). Begin with an initial oral dose of 1 mg/day (1/2 tablet). Prescribe only enough medication to last until the next visit (1 week later) to minimize risk of overdose.
3. Gradually increase the dose by 1 mg every 3–7 days until improvement of symptoms is noted and a maintenance dose can be established. It may take up to 6 weeks to obtain maximum therapeutic effect. Although the maximum dose is 10 mg/day, it is rarely necessary to exceed 4 mg/day.
4. After 2–3 months, gradually taper the dose by 1 mg every 3–7 days. Reinstitute therapy if the delusion recurs.
5. To avoid the extrapyramidal effects of restlessness and muscular stiffness caused by pimozide, give oral benzotropine mesylate (Cogentin) 2 mg t.i.d. p.r.n. or diphenhydramine (Benadryl) 10–25 mg p.o. t.i.d. p.r.n.

Alternative Therapy

1. For patients who do not tolerate pimozide, prescribe a less-potent antipsychotic agent such as oral trifluoperazine hydrochloride (Stelazine) 2–5 mg b.i.d.
2. For patients who are also depressed, or in whom pruritus and excoriations are present, pimozide may be used in combination with oral doxepin 100–300 mg/day, as the anticholinergic effects of doxepin often prevent the appearance of extrapyramidal side effects of pimozide.

Pitfalls

1. Proper diagnosis is critical to successful management. Psychiatric consultation is appropriate to ensure the diagnosis.
2. Pimozide can prolong the Q-T interval, and in the presence of underlying arrhythmia may result in sudden death although this is very unlikely in doses less than or equal to 4 mg/day. Perform a thorough history and physical, including ECG, prior to instituting pimozide therapy.
3. Pimozide may lower the seizure threshold, and is contraindicated in the presence of a history of seizure activity.

4. Pimozide has anticholinergic effects that may exacerbate glaucoma, constipation, and urinary retention.

BW

43

Dermatitis Herpetiformis

Dermatitis herpetiformis is a chronic, intensely pruritic disorder characterized by symmetrically distributed bullae or erosions, deposition of IgA in the dermal papillae, and evidence of gluten-sensitive enteropathy. Only 10% of patients experience remission. The therapeutic goal is control of pruritus and at least most of the skin lesions.

Initial Therapy

Following G6PD screening, the drug of choice is dapsone 100 mg/day. Expect a dramatic clinical response within 4–5 days. Re-evaluate the patient after 2 weeks, and increase dapsone to 200 mg/day if clinical improvement is inadequate. Check the CBC every 2 weeks as the dose is increased.

Subsequent Therapy

Continue the amount of dapsone required for clearing for 2 weeks, and then taper the drug by halving the dose every 2 weeks. Maintain the patient on the least amount of dapsone required for control of lesions. Once the appropriate dapsone dose is found, the CBC must be checked on a 6-month basis.

Alternative Therapy

1. Sulfapyridine, supplied in 500-mg tablets, may be used in an initial dose of 2 g in patients who cannot tolerate dapsone's side effects of nausea, lethargy, and depression. To determine the appropriate maintenance dose of

sulfapyridine, see the patient every 2 weeks. Control usually requires 1–4 g/day.

2. Combination therapy: If partial control is obtained on maximal doses of sulfapyridine (4 g/day), a small amount (25–50 mg) of dapsone may be added to the regimen.

3. Gluten-free diet: Because dermatitis herpetiformis is gluten dependent, many patients will respond to a gluten-free diet. Clinical response usually requires the patient to be on a rigid gluten-free diet for 6–12 months. To obtain dietary directions, refer the patient to a dietician. A successful dietary regimen requires an intelligent, highly motivated patient who dines at home. In appropriate patients, begin the gluten-free diet in combination with sulfone therapy.

Pitfalls

1. The diagnosis of dermatitis herpetiformis should be re-evaluated in patients who do not respond to appropriately administered sulfone therapy.

2. Screen patients prior to sulfone therapy for anemia and G6PD deficiency to avoid further anemia or severe drug-induced hemolysis.

3. Follow the CBC and reticulocyte count at regular intervals in all patients during adjustment of sulfone dose. Once treatment dose is established, these tests and a WBC need to be checked once or twice yearly.

BW

44

Dermatomyositis

Patients with dermatomyositis (DM) usually have multisystem involvement and therefore require a multidisciplinary approach to care and work-up. The incidence of underlying malignancy increases over age 40. In addition, some patients with DM display clinical features that overlap with systemic lupus erythematosus (SLE) and/or scleroderma. Management is also dictated by the patient's age group, as childhood cases exhibit a greater tendency for a more fulminant course, complicated by systemic necrotizing vasculitis. In addition, myositis followed by extensive calcinosis cutis is more common in children.

Initial Therapy

Systemic steroids: For adults, prednisone 60–100 mg/day in divided doses q.i.d. is standard therapy. In children, the initial dosage is 2 mg/kg/day, also in divided doses. Maintain this dose until objective and clinical signs of improvement in myositis occur. The total steroid dose then can be slowly decreased, with attempts made to adjust to a b.i.d. or q.d. regimen. However, DM usually cannot be controlled with q.o.d. steroids, and relapses are the rule when the steroid dose approaches 20–30 mg/day (1 mg/kg/day in children). Hence, cytotoxic agents (see below) may need to be added both as adjunctive therapy and for their steroid-sparing characteristics.

Alternate Therapy

Despite the above regimen, some cases of dermatomyositis may display a fulminant course. Such patients may benefit from either pulse therapy with megadoses of steroids (see Ch. 149 for guidelines) or plasmapheresis.

Ancillary Therapy

1. Cytotoxic agents: Give azathioprine 1–2 mg/kg/day or cyclophosphamide 1–2 mg/kg/day to reduce steroid requirements, and then taper slowly after the steroid dose is reduced to less than 20 mg/day.
2. Work-up for underlying malignancy is mandatory in adults with myositis with or without dermatitis. At least 25% will have carcinomas, and DM usually remits after complete removal of the offending malignancy.

Subsequent Therapy

1. Physical therapy, both passive and active, may be required to prevent contractures (in patients with and without calcinosis), but must be administered with care to patients with active myositis.
2. Ulcerations over pressure points owing to impaired movement or over sites of calcinosis can be recalcitrant to standard therapy. Vapor-permeable

dressings and adequate nutrition, with attention to water-soluble vitamin and mineral, intake may be helpful.

3. The dermatitis in DM is photosensitive, and sunscreens (SPF of 15 or greater to protect against both UVB and UVA) are indicated to prevent worsening of skin lesions. In patients with DM-SLE overlap syndromes, sunscreens also may prevent systemic flares.

4. For treatment of associated Raynaud's syndrome, see Chapter 151.

Pitfalls

1. The presence of potential side effects of systemic steroids, including GI hemorrhage, osteopenia, psychosis, cataracts, chemical diabetes, reactivation of latent tuberculosis, and increased frequency of infections, needs to be assessed repeatedly.

2. For the pitfalls associated with use of cytotoxic agents, see Appendix 7.

3. Calcinosis cutis can become very widespread, and can severely limit mobility, but when present signals a relatively quiescent or burnt-out stage of disease from which recovery may occur slowly over subsequent months to years.

4. Although an underlying malignancy may not be detectable in adult patients upon initial work-up, it may emerge at some later point. Hence, adult DM patients should be examined at regular intervals for the emergence of a previously occult neoplasm.

PE

45

Dermographism

Dermographism is a physical urticarial state characterized by whealing after stroking the skin or scratching. Most patients are mildly dermographic and require no therapy; some with severe pruritus and whealing, however, are said to have "symptomatic dermographism," and treatment of such individuals is appropriate.

Initial Therapy

Practical therapy is limited to the use of antihistamines alone or in combination. The therapeutic goal is to control pruritus and to limit whealing as much as possible. Patients may tolerate cutaneous lesions if symptoms are controlled. For any antihistamine prescribed, first determine the dose necessary to control pruritus and administer the medication in a manner that allows 24-hour antihistamine coverage. The following agents are preferred as initial therapy:

1. Hydroxyzine (Atarax) 25–50 mg b.i.d. to q.i.d. is often effective, but may cause drowsiness that resolves in most individuals after 5–7 days.
2. Terfenadine (Seldane) 60–120 mg b.i.d. to t.i.d. or astemizole (Hismanal) 10–20 mg/day are efficacious and do not cause drowsiness in most patients.

Subsequent Therapy

After symptoms have been controlled for 2 weeks, determine the least amount of medication necessary to meet the patient's therapeutic expectations. Attempt to wean the patient from medication every 2–3 months as the disorder spontaneously (and mysteriously) abates (in most individuals).

Alternative Therapy

1. Other antihistamines: Any other antihistamines may be tried, but many therapists use diphenhydramine (Benadryl) 25–50 mg t.i.d. to q.i.d. Marked drowsiness often limits the use of this agent.
2. Long-acting antihistamines: Many antihistamines are available in "long-acting" formulation. These have the advantage of less-frequent dosing.
3. Combinations of antihistamines.
    a. Hydroxyzine 25–50 t.i.d. to q.i.d with cyproheptadine (Periactin) 4 mg up to q.i.d.
    b. Cimetidine (Tagamet), an H_2 antagonist, 400 mg q.i.d. in combination with an H_1 blocker is useful in some individuals who do not respond to simpler regimens.

Pitfalls

1. The prescription of systemic steroids should be avoided. Although these agents often work, partial control of this benign process is preferable to the complications of steroid therapy.
2. Dermographism is rarely the presenting manifestation of systemic mastocytosis.

BW

46

Diabetic Dermopathy

Although diabetic dermopathy is strongly associated with diabetes, similar lesions can occur in other diseases accompanied by microangiopathy (e.g., rheumatoid arthritis). Because of their predominance on the shins, trauma is the presumed trigger factor, but the lesions themselves represent atrophic sequelae of earlier insults.

Initial Therapy

1. Diagnose and treat the underlying disease condition, usually diabetes. The skin lesions, however, do not change with treatment.
2. Instruct patients with dermopathy to avoid trauma; because of a frequently associated neuropathy, these patients are at increased risk for other trauma-induced lesions (e.g., malperforans ulcers).

Pitfalls

Diabetic dermopathy is associated with an increased incidence of neuropathy and retinopathy. Therefore, evaluate asymptomatic patients with dermopathy for these complications.

PE

47

Diaper Dermatitis

Diaper Rash

Diaper dermatitis is caused by maceration, irritants in stool and urine, altered pH, and microorganisms.

Initial Therapy

1. Regular prompt diaper changes: Instruct the parent or care-giver to clean the diaper area well and apply Desitin ointment. (Parents have usually done this but it needs to be reinforced.)
2. Nystatin ointment plus hydrocortisone 1% ointment mixed together applied with diaper changes.

Subsequent Therapy

1. Imidazole cream first followed by hydrocortisone 1% ointment with diaper changes.
2. Oral nystatin 100,000 U/ml t.i.d. if infection with *Candida* is suspected.
3. Encourage the use of superabsorbant disposable diapers or a diaper service.

Pitfalls

1. Look for associated bacterial infection and treat.
2. Metabolic diseases and histiocytosis X may present as a diaper dermatitis.
3. Viral exanthems (hand, foot, and mouth; varicella) may begin and remain in the diaper area.

TB

48

Discoid Lupus Erythematosus

Discoid lupus erythematosus (DLE) typically is a light-sensitive dermatosis that occurs as an isolated disease in over 95% of cases. Rarely, DLE will progress to systemic lupus erythematosus (SLE). However, patients with SLE may have discoid skin lesions. The primary goal of therapy is to prevent or minimize disfigurement.

Initial Therapy

1. Topical steroids: Prescribe a superpotent steroid cream (see Appendix 1), to be applied b.i.d. to areas of active disease. (To minimize the potential atrophogenic side effects of topical steroids to facial lesions, discontinue this therapy or change to a nonatrophogenic, low-potency preparation as soon as a response occurs, or after a maximum of 2 weeks.)
2. Intralesional steroids: Intralesional triamcinolone acetonide (Kenalog) diluted 1 : 1 with lidocaine 1% (final concentration 5 mg/cc) can be administered to active lesions or advancing edges of discoid lesions. Do not perform this therapy more often than once every 3–4 weeks to minimize atrophy.

Alternative Therapy

1. Antimalarials may be helpful in patients who are either photosensitive or unresponsive to steroid therapy. Hydroxychloroquine (Plaquenil) 200 mg b.i.d. usually results in a gradual reduction of inflammation over 3 months. If a good response has occurred, the dose can be lowered to 200 mg/day indefinitely. If only a partial response has occurred, add quinacrine (Atabrine) 100 mg/day for 1–3 months to the hydroxychloroquine regimen.
2. Systemic steroids sometimes are effective for patients in whom antimalarials are contraindicated. A typical regimen consists of prednisone 40 mg q.a.m. for 2–3 weeks, followed by tapering if a response occurs. A more prolonged 4–6 week course with tapering may be used if the response is slow.
3. If the response to antimalarials is unsatisfactory, clofazimine (Lamprene) 100 mg b.i.d. can be tried alone or in conjunction with antimalarials.
4. Azathioprine (Imuran), 50–100 mg/day, decreasing to 25–50 mg/day after a response is observed, has been reported to be helpful for refractory cases of DLE that did not respond to antimalarials.

Subsequent Therapy and Work-Up

1. All patients with DLE should use a sunscreen (SPF 15 or greater), as excessive sun exposure can result in further spread or reactivation of quiescent disease. Moreover, the depigmented areas of DLE are at greater risk for the development of actinically induced malignancies.
2. Camouflage techniques are particularly helpful in blacks with DLE. Several lines of cosmetics are designed to mask pigmentary abnormalities such as those in DLE (e.g., Dermablend, Covermark, Lydia O'Leary). However, these cosmetics often are available only in cosmetic departments of large department stores.
3. About 20% of patients with DLE have a positive ANA (titer $\geq 1 : 40$), and a comparable percent may have anti-single-stranded DNA antibodies (ssDNA). Evaluate these patients for possible SLE, including a baseline LFT and renal function study.
4. All patients with DLE should have laboratory parameters checked for the development of SLE at approximately yearly intervals.

Pitfalls

1. Topical and intralesional steroids are potentially atrophogenic and can themselves produce pigmentary abnormalities. Prolonged or excessive usage can worsen the disfigurement in DLE.
2. Antimalarials can produce retinal toxicity, and patients on this form of therapy should be assessed by an ophthalmologist at 6-month intervals.
3. Antimalarials can cause acute hemolysis in G6PD-deficient patients; hence, a screen for this enzyme must be obtained prior to initiation of therapy.
4. Biologically aggressive squamous cell carcinomas can occur in old scars of DLE (as in any other cutaneous scarring process). Thus, even patients with quiescent disease need to be examined regularly for the presence of neoplastic lesions.
5. Quinacrine (Atabrine) can cause a lemon-yellow discoloration of the skin.
6. Clofazimine (Lamprene) produces generalized hyperpigmentation in almost 100% of patients, and ichthyosis in up to 50% of patients.
7. The side effects of azathioprine (Imuran) are described in Appendix 7.

PE

49

Drug Eruptions

Drugs cause a variety of cutaneous reactions. Therapy of the most common of these, the "moribilliform" or measle-like pattern, is discussed here. Other specific drug-induced disorders such as urticaria, erythema multiforme, toxic epidermal necrolysis, and phototoxicity are discussed in other chapters.

Initial Therapy

1. Discontinue the offending drug. If patients are on multiple medications and definite causal identification is not possible, attempt to identify the most likely offending drug and discontinue it and all unnecessary drugs. Use alternative, nonchemically related agents. In most cases, the cutaneous reaction will resolve in 2–5 days without therapy. Some patients, however, may require topical or systemic therapy to control the bothersome pruritus that may accompany the reaction.

   If no other therapeutic alternatives are possible, the clinicians may elect to continue the offending drug despite the eruption, as many cases will resolve. Watch for serum sickness, progression to erythroderma, exfoliation, erythema multiforme, or toxic epidermal necrolysis.
2. Antihistamines, such as hydroxyzine 25–50 mg t.i.d. or q.i.d., are often adequate.
2. Topical therapy with bland agents and hydration are helpful. Instruct the patient to soak in a warm bath for 10–15 minutes b.i.d. or t.i.d. Oilated colloidal oatmeal (Aveeno) may be added. Application of an emollient (e.g., Eucerin, Aquaphor) should follow each bath.
4. If aggressive hydration and application of emollients is unrealistic, application of a medium-potency fluorinated steroid ointment b.i.d. or t.i.d. is helpful. Expect resolution of the process in 2–5 days.

Alternative Therapy

In rare cases, the cutaneous reaction may be so severe as to require systemic steroids. If necessary, treat with prednisone using a 10-day tapering-dose regimen beginning at 40–60 mg/day for adults, and 1–

2 mg/kg/day for children. Treat at the highest steroid dose for 4–5 days before tapering.

Pitfalls

1. If the cutaneous reaction does not resolve as expected, consider another diagnosis or the possibility that the offending agent has not been discontinued.
2. Look for liver, renal, and hematologic abnormalities, particularly if drugs such as dilantin and allopurinol are possible offenders.
3. In patients with renal or hepatic insufficiency, drug clearance may be impaired and the rash may persist longer than 3–5 days after discontinuation.
4. Look for mononucleosis if the offender is a semisynthetic penicillin (especially ampicillin).
5. A morbilliform rash may rarely be a prodrome of toxic epidermal necrolysis. Check for skin tenderness and bullous lesions.

BW

50

Eczemas

Nummular Eczemas

Eczema is an all-inclusive term for dermatitis of diverse origin, including atopic dermatitis, dyshidrotic eczema, hand eczema, seborrheic dermatitis, and stasis dermatitis (see appropriate chapters for descriptions of therapy for these disease entities). Nummular eczema is an inflammatory disorder consisting of one or more coin-shaped patches, usually on the legs, but not uncommonly on the arms and trunk, as well. Older age groups are affected predominantly, and individuals with chronic dry skin and/or atopies also are preferentially affected.

Initial Therapy

1. Prescribe an intermediate-potency steroid cream to be applied in a thin film b.i.d. (see Appendix 1). The rash should disappear slowly over 1–3 weeks.
2. General measures:
   a. Hydration of the skin with a water-in-oil ointment (e.g., Aquaphor, Eucerin) applied q.d. immediately after bathing may be helpful.
   b. Discourage excessive bathing (more than once a day), especially during winter months.
   c. Encourage bathing in cool-to-tepid water and the use of mild soaps (e.g., Dove (avoid Ivory)). Soap should not be applied to the lesions, if possible.
   d. Calamine or other drying lotions are to be avoided.
   e. Woolen or acrylic clothing and blankets should be avoided.

Alternative Therapy

1. Recalcitrant cases may be treated with steroids plus a topical tar preparation (e.g., Fototar) applied q.d. to the rash only.
2. A course of systemic antibiotics (e.g., erythromycin or dicloxacillin 250 mg t.i.d.) may help some recalcitrant cases.
3. Antihistamines (e.g., hydroxyzine 25–50 mg or doxepin 25 mg), especially at bedtime, may be useful in cases in which pruritus is severe.
4. A course of systemic steroids (e.g., intramuscular triamcinalone acetonide (Kenalog) 40 mg stat or prednisone) in a tapering 10-day schedule should be reserved only for the most stubborn cases.

Pitfalls

1. Consider tinea corporis, contact dermatitis, parapsoriasis, and mycosis fungoides in any recalcitrant case. A KOH preparation is indicated if scale or an active border is present.
2. The side effects of systemic steroids are discussed in Appendix 5.

PE

51

Ecthyma Gangrenosum

Although lesions of ecthyma gangrenosum (EG) may occur in the absence of sepsis, most cases are life threatening owing to gram-negative sepsis (usually, but not invariably, *P. aeruginosa*), and are often best managed in an intensive care unit with the assistance of experts in infectious disease.

Initial Therapy

For severe cases, an aminoglycoside, gentamicin, or tobramycin 1.5 mg/kg q.8h. and carbenicillin 300–900 mg/kg/day, piperacillin or ticarcillin 2–3 g q.4h. by intravenous infusion are the preferred therapy. Amikacin can be substituted for gentamicin or tobramycin. For more limited disease, gentamicin alone, in lower doses (e.g., 5 mg/kg/day), may suffice.

Ancillary Therapy

Therapy may be needed for associated disseminated intravascular coagulation and/or shock.

Alternative Therapy

1. Intravenous chloramphenicol can be substituted for carbenicillin in penicillin-allergic individuals, depending on microbial sensitivities.
2. Intravenous third-generation cephalosporins or polymyxin B can be substituted for aminoglycosides in allergic patients, or in patients with renal or otic contraindications to the use of aminoglycoside drugs.

Pitfalls

1. *Pseudomonas* is the prototypic cause, but not the only cause, of EG. EG-like lesions occur with sepsis owing to a wide variety of organisms, including *Candida*.

2. Assess patients with EG for the presence of an underlying immunodeficiency state (e.g., leukemia, if previously undiagnosed).
3. Immunosuppressed patients are particularly at risk for gram-negative sepsis, mandating extra precautions and aggressive responses to early signs of sepsis.
4. *Pseudomonas* can be harbored in many places in a hospital setting (e.g., sinks, flower vases, topical creams and ointments, toilets, and nebulizers).
5. Aminoglycosides cause irreversible ototoxicity and nephrotoxicity in a dose-dependent fashion. Blood levels of drug must be monitored, and both renal and auditory function regularly assessed.

PE

52

Eosinophilic Fasciitis

Eosinophilic fasciitis is distinguished from scleroderma by its acute onset, its lack of acral or visceral involvement, its tendency to spontaneously remit after 2–5 years, and its exquisite responsiveness to systemic corticosteroid therapy.

Initial Therapy

1. Prednisone 20–30 mg/day, given in a single morning dose, will clear the inflammatory phase, but higher doses (20–30 mg b.i.d.) are required to control any associated fibrosis. After improvement in either or both manifestations, slowly taper therapy over 6–12 months to a maintenance dose of 5 mg/day, and finally, switch to 10 mg q.o.d.
2. Include in the initial work-up a skin biopsy that extends to the muscle fascia; total eosinophil count; serum protein and immunoelectrophoresis; serum eosinophil chemotactic factor (if available); and serial determinations of the ESR.

Alternative Therapy

1. Cimetidine 400 mg q.i.d. has been reported to reverse both the inflammation and induration in eosinophilic fasciitis.

2. Hydroxychloroquine (Plaquenil) 200 mg b.i.d. may be useful for induration, particularly for patients who cannot receive higher doses of systemic
   steroids.
3. Aspirin 6–8 tablets/day may be helpful for the inflammatory phase, particularly if steroids are contraindicated.
4. P-Aminobenzoic acid (PABA, Potaba) 2 g q.i.d. reportedly has helped
   some patients with persistent induration.

Pitfalls

1. Eosinophilic fasciitis must be distinguished from scleroderma. Recognition
   is important because therapy and prognosis are radically different.
2. Side effects of systemic steroids are described in Appendix 5.
3. Side effects of antimalarials are described in Chapter 48.
4. Cimetidine can produce signs of feminization (e.g., gynecomastia) and a
   host of other side effects, including allergic cutaneous vasculitis.

PE

53

Epidermal Nevus

Therapy is usually purely for cosmetic reasons.

Initial Therapy

1. The overlying hyperkeratosis may be treated with topical lactic acid (Lac-
   Hydrin, LactiCare), salicylic acid (Keralyt Gel), or retinoic acid preparations, applied q.d. immediately after bathing.
2. For large, systematized, and/or inflammatory lesions, oral retinoids (as for
   ichthyosis; see Ch. 94) may be considered.
3. Refer patients with epidermal nevi for baseline and, if indicated, repeated
   neurologic and orthopedic evaluations to detect associated CNS and musculoskeletal defects (epidermal nevus syndrome).

Alternative Therapy

Adequate surgical management of epidermal nevi usually involves
the removal or destruction of a significant portion of subjacent der-

mis. Scarring, therefore, may result. Initially, attempt cryotherapy. If this fails, dermabrasion, deep shaving, or surgical excision may be considered.

Pitfalls

1. The complications of oral retinoids are discussed in Appendix 1.
2. Surgical removal of epidermal nevi often results in scarring, and patients should be appropriately counselled.

TB

54

Epidermolysis Bullosa: General Guidelines

Epidermolysis bullosa (EB) is a heterogeneous group of inherited mechanobullous diseases that is constantly expanding. Three basic forms are recognized, based on the electron microscopic level of the blister formation. There are several basic principles in the management of all cases of EB; they are outlined below. Specific therapy for each group is described in the appropriate chapter.

Basic Therapeutic Principles

1. Establishing the diagnosis: There is tremendous clinical overlap, so virtually all cases require electron microscopy or immunofluorescent mapping for correct diagnosis. This is critical for therapy, genetic counselling, and prognosis.
2. Genetic counselling: Since these diseases are inherited, genetic counselling is essential. Prenatal diagnosis via fetal biopsy is available for patients in whom previous pregnancies resulted in severely affected children.
3. Family education: Some forms of EB are devastating, and demand a significant commitment on the part of the patient, the family, and health care providers. The Dystrophic Epidermolysis Bullosa Research Associa-

tion of America (DEBRA) (Kings County Medial Center, 451 Clarkson Avenue, Bldg. E, 6th Floor, #E6101, Brooklyn, NY 11203; telephone (718)774-8700) has been a pioneer patient support and education group. Every family with severely affected children should contact this group for support and continual education.

4. Trauma: Even very minor trauma induces lesions. Efforts to reduce trauma by protection and lubrication are essential to care.

5. Infection: Healing is diminished by secondary infection of skin lesions, usually by *S. aureus* or β-hemolytic streptococci. Prophylactic use of antibacterial ointments, specifically mupirocin (Bactroban), has been of great help. When obvious infection occurs, administer an oral semisynthetic penicillin (dicloxacillin) or a first-generation cephalosporin. Perform cultures, especially in those EB patients who have received multiple courses of systemic antibiotics, as antibiotic resistance may occur. Prophylactic antibiotics may be considered in those patients with frequent infections.

6. Blister care: The normal skin forming the roof of the blister should be left on as long as possible; it is the optimal biologic dressing. If the hydrostatic pressure of the fluid in the blister tends to increase its size, open the blister and drain the fluid. If a blister becomes infected, drain it and remove the roof.

TB

55

Epidermolysis Bullosa Aquisita

Epidermolysis bullosa aquisita (EBA) is the only non-hereditary form of epidermolysis bullosa. The original reports of EBA described only noninflammatory acquired cases resembling inherited dystrophic epidermolysis bullosa. Now it is recognized that EBA may also present as an inflammatory bullous disorder clinically similar to bullous pemphigoid, cicatricial pemphigoid, or porphyria cutanea tarda. Diagnosis is confirmed by special immunofluorescent studies or electron microscopy. Therapy is generally difficult, and most patients have a chronic progressive disorder lasting many years. The aggressiveness of treatment should correlate with the severity of disease. No universally effective therapy has been found for those patients with the classic disorder of skin fragility and noninflammatory lesions.

Initial Therapy

1. For patients with localized, nonmucosal, noninflammatory EBA, topical management is the initial therapy. More aggressive treatment is rarely indicated, as potentially effective therapies have significant side effects.
   a. Protect the affected area with soft dressings to prevent trauma.
   b. Prescribe antibacterial emollients (bacitracin or mupirocin ointment) to reduce friction and prevent secondary infection.
   c. Try intermediate-potency to superpotent topical steroids.
2. For patients with localized disease of the mucosa, face, or genitalia, and for generalized inflammatory disease, administer systemic therapy as suggested for bullous pemphigoid (see Ch. 22).
   a. Prednisone 1–2 mg/kg in divided doses is suggested, but results vary from total resolution to no response.
   b. Dapsone has been found to be beneficial in patients who had an intense dermal polymorphonuclear leukocyte infiltrate.

Subsequent Therapy

1. If the patient responds to systemic steroids, the dose should be slowly tapered. The use of antimetabolites (cyclophosphamide or azathioprine) as steroid-sparing agents has not been useful to date. Unfortunately, many patients require dosages of systemic steroids that lead to long-term complications.
2. Patients failing to respond to systemic steroids who have severe, progressive disease may be considered for low-dose cyclosporin A (4–6 mg/kg).
3. Plasmapheresis has been useful in one patient, and its use should be considered in severe cases with measurable titers of circulating autoantibody. Autoantibody titers may fall with no clinical improvement, however.

Pitfalls

1. The major pitfall is not recognizing EBA. Direct immunofluorescence is essential in the evaluation of most bullous eruptions.
2. The complications of systemic steroids are in Appendix 5. For complications of dapsone therapy, see Chapter 84, Hansen's Disease.

3. Cyclosporin A has many side effects, and its prescription should be restricted to physicians with experience with this drug. Nephrotoxicity, dose-dependent elevation of LFTs, immunosuppression, gingival hypertrophy, hypertrichosis, and neurologic side effects have all been reported. Toxic side effects are dose dependent, and can be reduced by monitoring blood levels.
4. Mucous membranes are often severely affected. The appropriate specialist (ophthalmologist, gastroenterologist, urologist, or gynecologist) should be consulted when there is significant involvement of the mucosal surfaces.

TB

56

Epidermolysis Bullosa, Dystrophic

Dominant Dystrophic Epidermolysis Bullosa • Recessive Dystrophic Epidermolysis Bullosa

At least six forms of dystrophic epidermolysis bullosa (EB) occur. Patients having dominantly inherited forms tend to do better, and although scarring occurs, this subgroup does fairly well and may improve considerably with age. The generalized recessive dystrophic type (RDEB) is often a devastating progressive disease with severe morbidity.

Initial Therapy

1. Many patients with RDEB respond to oral phenytoin, with about a 50% decrease in blistering. Follow blood levels and maintain at approximately 8 mg/L.
2. Aggressive local care with whirlpools, gentle cleansing with mild antibacterial soaps (chlorhexidine 3%), use of emollient antibacterial ointments

(mupirocin, silver sulfadiazine, bacitracin), and careful application of dressings (Exudry) is essential. Extensive and detailed instructions on these techniques can be found in *Advances in Dermatology* 3:99–120 (1988). DEBRA (see Ch. 54) may also help families learn these techniques. The manufacturer of mupirocin ointment has provided the ointment without charge in the amounts these patients require.

3. For the mitis type of RDEB, but not the severe type, vitamin E (α-tocopherol) 1,600 U/day may be useful.

Subsequent Therapy

1. The management of RDEB requires a team approach. In addition to skin care, nutritional support, physical therapy, psychological support, and good dental care are all essential. Patients should be referred to specialists in each of these fields for regular visits. Ocular, GI tract, GU tract, and respiratory tract complications often occur, usually as a result of scarring. Specialists may need to be consulted.

2. Malnutrition and anemia are common. Caloric needs are increased by constant skin and blood loss. Transfusion may be required.

3. Any nonhealing ulcer or lesion appearing at the edge of a nonhealing ulcer should be carefully evaluated for the possibility of squamous cell carcinoma.

4. Repeated surgical procedures may be required to release mitten hands and keep digits functional.

5. Regular immunizations should be given.

Pitfalls

1. Phenytoin may cause a severe hypersensitivity syndrome resembling infectious mononucleosis. Gingival hyperplasia is common.

2. Bacitracin should be applied only to localized areas, as systemic absorption and potential nephrotoxicity or ototoxicity may occur.

3. Silver sulfadiazine can cause hyperosmotic coma in infants, and should not be used in neonates or small infants, except in limited areas.

4. Caution must be used when applying semipermeable dressings, as infection may be enhanced beneath them in this setting. Also, when removed, the adherent dressing may tear off the fragile epidermis. The thicker dressings (Duoderm, Restore) may occasionally be useful on chronically traumatized areas such as the elbows or knees, whereas the transparent dressings give better visualization of the underlying erosions and are better suited for other less traumatized areas. The high cost of these dressings precludes their widespread or frequent use in these patients, and more economical

alternatives (antibiotic ointments plus Exudry or Telfa) have been effective.

TB

57

Epidermolysis Bullosa, Junctional

At least five forms of junctional epidermolysis bullosa (JEB) are recognized. All are autosomally recessively inherited. Involvement may be mild (generalized atrophic, localized, and inverse types) or severe (Herlitz and gravis types). Systemic involvement may occur. Pyloric atresia is uniquely associated with JEB. One variant of JEB, cicatricial type, may develop scarring similar to that in patients with recessive dystrophic EB.

Initial Therapy

1. Local care with protection, ointments (mupirocin, silver sulfadiazine or bacitracin), and dressings (Exudry) secured with wraps. Semipermeable dressings may be used, but they may tear off fragile epithelium when removed. Excellent management guidelines for the care of severely affected JEB patients are given in *Advances in Dermatology* 3:99–120, 1988.
2. Initial data suggest that generalized atrophic benign JEB, but not severe (Herlitz type) JEB, responds to oral phenytoin. Blood levels of phenytoin must be monitored and maintained at approximately 8 mg/L.

Subsequent Therapy

1. Children with JEB have hypoplastic enamel and resultant premature caries of both deciduous and permanent teeth. A skilled pediatric dentist must be a part of the health care team.
2. Bladder and ureteral involvement may rarely occur in JEB, leading to hydronephrosis. This should be watched for.

3. Facial erosions, characteristic of JEB and difficult to heal, may be treated with epidermal autografts if conservative methods fail (refer to *Archives of Dermatology* 124:732, 1988).

Pitfalls

1. At birth, it may be difficult to determine which form of JEB the child has. A trial of phenytoin is reasonable in progressive disease, as is an attempt with systemic steroid therapy.
2. Phenytoin may cause a severe hypersensitivity syndrome resembling infectious mononucleosis. Gingival hyperplasia is common.
3. Bacitracin should be applied only to localized areas, as systemic absorption and potential nephrotoxicity or ototoxicity may occur.
4. Caution must be used when applying semipermeable dressings, as infection may be enhanced beneath them in this setting.

TB

58

Epidermolysis Bullosa Simplex

At least five subtypes of epidermolysis bullosa simplex (EB simplex) are recognized. All forms are inherited by autosomal dominance. This disease may be generalized and severe (EB herpetiformis of Dowling-Meara), generalized and mild to moderate (Koebner type), or localized to the acral areas (Weber-Cockayne type). Scarring in general does not occur except when lesions become secondarily infected. Because life-threatening complications, scarring, and mucosal involvement are minimal or absent, supportive therapy is usually adequate.

LOCALIZED TYPE

Initial Therapy

1. Protection and lubrication.
2. Reduction of sweating by lowering the ambient temperature and/or performance of physical tasks during cooler times of the year.

3. Reduction of sweating of the palms and soles with aluminum chloride solutions (Drysol 20%, Xerac AC 6.25%) applied q.h.s. with occlusion until sweating is decreased. Glutaraldehyde 10% solution may also be used, but the skin will be stained and contact sensitization may occur (see Ch. 93, Hyperhidrosis).

GENERALIZED TYPE

Initial Therapy

1. Reduction of sweating by lowering the ambient temperature (except perhaps in Dowling-Meara type, where cold may worsen blistering).
2. Lubrication of the skin and prevention of secondary infection with bacitracin or mupirocin ointment.

TB

59

Erythema Annulare Centrifugum

Gyrate Erythemas • Figurate Erythemas • Migratory Erythemas

Gyrate erythemas are reactive processes. The most important aspect of their therapy is to search for the underlying cause. This discussion does not apply to the following members of the erythema group: erythema gyratum repens, which is a rare form almost universally associated with internal malignancy; erythema chronicum migrans, which is the primary stage of Lyme disease (see Ch. 60); erythema marginatum, which occurs with acute rheumatic fever; and necrolytic migratory erythema, which is associated with a glucagon-secreting tumor (see Ch. 124).

Initial Therapy

1. Search for an underlying cause, specifically tinea pedis or cruris. A complete physical examination is required, especially if tinea is not found, to rule out an underlying malignancy.
2. If tinea is found, best results are obtained with a 6–8-week course of oral griseofulvin or ketaconazole. Topical antifungals may not adequately reduce the tinea for the gyrate erythema to clear.
3. Systemic corticosteroids will improve most cases, but should only be administered for short periods, and only after a search for an underlying cause has been performed. Occasionally, empiric therapy with an antifungal or anticandidal agent, even in the absence of infections, will lead to clearing.

Pitfalls

1. Failure to evaluate and re-evaluate for an underlying cause.
2. Lupus erythematosus and rarely cutaneous T cell lymphoma may present as a gyrate erythema. A biopsy is indicated in all but the most classic cases.

TB

60

Erythema Chronicum Migrans

Primary Lyme Disease

Initial Therapy

1. Oral tetracycline 250 mg q.i.d. for 10–21 days or doxycycline 100 mg b.i.d. in adults; in children over 8 years of age, tetracycline 40 mg/kg/day in four divided doses, or
2. Oral penicillin V 500 mg q.i.d. for 10–21 days (for adults allergic to tetracycline); or 50 mg/kg/day in four divided doses in children 8 years of age and under.

Alternative Therapy

Although there are no studies to support its use in early Lyme disease, ceftriaxone has been shown to be effective in late Lyme disease refractory to penicillin therapy. The causative spirochete is extremely sensitive to this agent, and it may be the most effective agent in those cases failing to respond to initial tetracycline therapy. This agent must be given parenterally.

Subsequent Therapy

Regular follow-up of these patients for potential cardiac, neurologic, or arthritic sequelae is important. These sequelae can be treated with high-dose parenteral penicillin or ceftriaxone.

Pitfall

Erythema chronicum migrans is a clinical diagnosis, as serologic testing (as in primary syphilis) may be negative at this stage. Given the benign nature of the treatment and the severity of potential sequelae, refer the patient for consultation and treat early if this diagnosis is entertained.

TB

61

Erythema Elevatum Diutinum

Extracellular Cholesterosis

Initial Therapy

Oral dapsone 50–100 mg q.d. is the preferred initial therapy.

Alternative Therapy

Intralesional triamcinolone acetonide 2.5–5 mg/cc may be used if there are few lesions.

Subsequent Therapy

1. Prophylactic oral penicillin or erythromycin 250 mg/day may help to reduce lesions and supplement the above therapy.
2. In patients failing to respond to low-dose dapsone, the dosage may be increased to a maximum of 200 mg/day.

Pitfalls

For side effects of dapsone therapy, see Chapter 84, Hansen's Disease. Check the G6PD level before instituting treatment, and follow the CBC.

TB

62

Erythema Multiforme

The presence of annular lesions, often acrally distributed, with a central target or bulla, is characteristic of erythema multiforme (EM). Atypical forms with urticarial plaques or oral lesions alone, however, can present diagnostic dilemmas. Therapy is generally not required or helpful for EM minor (limited to skin and/or one mucosal surface without systemic symptoms), which is a self-limited process. EM major (Stevens–Johnson syndrome), however, requires in-patient management because of significant systemic symptoms and involvement of one or more mucosal surfaces. Unfortunately, specific therapy does not exist, and administration of systemic steroids may actually cause unanticipated complications. Fortunately, like EM minor, the disease is self-limited regardless of severity.

Initial Therapy

1. For bullous skin lesions, Domeboro compresses (1 packet dissolved in 1 pt tap water) applied b.i.d. for 20 minutes followed by applications of silver sulfadiazine (Silvadene) cream b.i.d. Note: Mafenide acetate (Sulfamy-

lon) should be avoided, as it can exacerbate or precipitate sulfonamide-induced EM.

2. For systemic oral lesions, an antiseptic mouthwash or hydrogen peroxide 30%, diluted 1 : 9, should be used t.i.d.

3. For ocular lesions, the most devastating potential complication of Stevens-Johnson syndrome, refer the patient to an ophthalmologist. There currently is no evidence that either systemic or intraocular steroids can prevent progression of ocular disease. Note: Avoid sulfa-containing eyedrops for the reasons given above.

4. Parenteral fluid replacement may be needed for patients with extensive erosions, particularly if oral lesions compromise fluid intake. Monitor fluid requirements by observing blood pressure, urine output, daily weights, and assessment of central venous pressure, if necessary.

Ancillary Therapy

1. EM is triggered by either infection (most commonly either type I or II herpes simplex, but also *M. pneumoniae* and a variety of other organisms) or drugs. Therefore, a search for the underlying cause is indicated. Although therapy for coexistent or antecedent herpes infections (e.g., with acyclovir) will not impact on the course of an individual episode of EM, suppressive therapy with acyclovir may prevent subsequent attacks. Implement treatment of other infectious causes because rarely epidemics of EM follow transmission of pathogens to other individuals.

2. Patients receiving sulfonamides, antiepileptics, analgesics, or antibiotics are suspect for having drug-induced disease. Discontinue the offending agent and monitor the patient for progression to toxic epidermal necrolysis (a rare event, not occurring after infection-related disease). Cutaneous tenderness and widespread bulla formation (epidermolysis) are important clues. Immediate skin biopsy with frozen sections is indicated, and therapy then becomes that for toxic epidermal necrolysis (see Ch. 178).

3. Monitor for sepsis. With a compromised skin barrier, patients with bullous EM are prone to become septic. However, prophylactic antibiotics are not routinely indicated.

Pitfalls

1. As described above, drug-induced EM rarely may progress to toxic epidermal necrolysis.

2. There is a tendency for recurrent EM in patients with recurrent herpes simplex infections. Prophylactic acyclovir 200–600 mg/day may prevent flares of both herpes and resultant episodes of EM.

3. If the patient was treated with systemic steroids before being seen, the possibility that complications of steroid therapy (e.g., sepsis) are already present must be considered.

PE

63

Erythema Nodosum

Erythema nodosum is a reactive inflammatory panniculitis produced by multiple agents and underlying conditions. The most important consideration in the management of erythema nodosum is to determine the cause and treat it.

Initial Therapy

1. Bed rest with elevation, elastic stockings, and/or an Ace wrap may be all that is required for relief in 2–3 days.
2. Aspirin or NSAIDs to tolerance may be added for analgesic effect and to enhance resolution.

Alternative Therapy

1. Oral potassium iodide (SSKI) 300 mg (5–6 drops) t.i.d. initially, increased by 1 drop/dose/day to resolution, is often dramatically beneficial. The patient is maintained on the dose adequate for response for a total of 3 weeks.
2. Indomethacin 25–50 mg t.i.d. may be effective.

Subsequent Therapy

INITIAL POSITIVE RESPONSE

Do not discontinue therapy too rapidly in those patients responding to the above treatments. Continuation of therapy for 2–3 weeks reduces recurrences.

FAILURE TO RESPOND TO THE ABOVE TREATMENTS

1. Colchicine 0.6–1.2 mg b.i.d.
2. Intralesional triamcinolone acetonide (Kenalog) 5 mg/cc to the center of individual lesions will cause them to resolve. This is good treatment if there are few lesions.
3. Because many cases are poststreptococcal, an empiric trial of oral penicillin or erythromycin 250 mg q.i.d. may be attempted.
4. Systemic corticosteroids in moderate doses (20–40 mg/day) will clear most cases. This therapy can only be used after the underlying cause has been identified and, if infectious, has been treated appropriately. Systemic steroids are contraindicated in those cases triggered by systemic fungal infections or tuberculosis.

Pitfalls

1. The major pitfall is failure to identify the underlying cause.
2. Clinically erythema nodosum and other panniculitides may not be easy to differentiate. If there is any question an excisional biopsy, including adequate subcutaneous fat, is required.

TB

64

Erythrasma

Initial Therapy

Topical erythromycin 2% solution or clindamycin 1% solution b.i.d. for 2–3 weeks is often curative.

Alternative Therapy

1. A topical imidazole cream applied b.i.d. for 4 weeks.
2. Oral erythromycin or tetracycline 250 mg q.i.d. for 7–10 days.

Pitfalls

Tinea versicolor of the groin is clinically very similar to erythrasma. Perform a KOH preparation to rule out tinea versicolor and tinea cruris.

TB

65

Erythromelalgia

Erythermalgia

Erythromelalgia is a rare syndrome characterized by pain in the distal extremities associated with increased blood flow and skin temperature. It can be incapacitating, and usually afflicts the lower extremities, although the upper extremities can be involved as well.

Initial Therapy

1. Acetylsalicylic acid (aspirin) 3 g/day initially is the treatment of choice, although it is not effective in all cases. After a response is achieved, the dose can be tapered slowly to the level that controls symptoms.
2. β-blockers can be helpful in cases not responding to aspirin, or in addition to aspirin. Begin with propanalol 20 mg t.i.d. and slowly increase the dose as tolerated until symptoms are controlled.

Alternative Therapy

1. Other NSAIDs (e.g., naproxen, ibuprofen) may be helpful in cases that fail to respond to aspirin and/or β-blockers.
2. Systemic steroids and chemotherapeutic agents have helped some patients.
3. Phlebotomy has helped some patients with erythromelalgia associated with polycythemia vera (see below).
4. Intravenous or subcutaneous heparin has helped some patients with dem-

onstrated thrombotic disease (e.g., as in some myeloproliferative disorders).

Ancillary Therapy

1. Point out the need to avoid hot environments; cool compresses or ice baths may abort individual episodes.
2. A work-up to rule out underlying disease is imperative; most commonly, polycythemia vera, essential hypertension, and systemic lupus erythematosus have been associated with erythromelalgia. However, there also appears to be an association with diabetes, gout, syphilis, rheumatoid arthritis, and multiple sclerosis.
3. Certain drugs and chemicals, including nicotine, bromocriptine, calcium channel blockers, and dopamine agonists, can exacerbate erythromelalgia. Dietary additives, such as cyclamates, tartrazine, and caffeine, may be provocative in individual cases.
4. Biofeedback techniques and relaxation exercises can reduce the frequency and severity of attacks.
5. Elevation of the legs, including raising the foot of the bed, can be helpful.

Pitfalls

1. Patients with erythromelalgia need a thorough work-up for underlying precipitating disease and/or drug etiology.
2. Patients receiving β-blockers should be warned to avoid substantial amounts of epinephrine (e.g., in local anesthetics) because of the potential for unrestricted α-adrenergic stimulation, leading to severe hypertension.

PE

66

Erythropoietic Protoporphyria

Initial Therapy

1. Oral β-carotene 60–180 mg/day (2 to 6 capsules) indefinitely. The dose is adjusted to maintain serum carotene levels above 400 μg/100 ml and ideally between 600 and 800 μg/100 ml.

2. Patients must use sun protection, even for sunlight exposure through window glass. Physical barrier protection (hat, gloves, clothes, zinc oxide paste) is required, as the active wavelengths are in the 400–410-nm (Soret band) range.

Subsequent Therapy

1. The maximum benefit from β-carotene therapy is seen after 1–3 months of treatment.
2. LFTs must be performed regularly to detect hepatic damage from erythropoietic protoporphyria. These patients may also develop gallstones, therefore a baseline sonogram of the gallbladder is indicated. If hepatic failure develops, some benefit may be gained by combined cholestyramine (12 g q.i.d.) and vitamin E (100 U/day).

Pitfalls

1. Nonopaque sunscreens are of no benefit. Physical barriers must be used. Loose-weave cotton or acrylic fibers allow some light to penetrate through the fabric and thus are to be avoided.
2. β-carotene colors the skin yellow, especially where the stratum corneum is thick (palms and soles), or where β-carotene is excreted onto the skin surface via sebaceous secretions (e.g., the face).
3. Less commonly, β-carotene will cause mild diarrhea or GI distress.

TB

67

Erythroplasia of Queyrat

Erythroplasia of Queyrat is squamous cell carcinoma in situ of the glans penis.

Initial Therapy

Prescribe 5-fluorouracil (5-FU) 5% cream to be applied b.i.d. with foreskin or condom occlusion for 3–4 weeks. Expect intense erosion and moderate discomfort.

Alternative Therapy

1. Cryotherapy using liquid nitrogen spray with local anesthesia and thermocouple control may be of benefit.
2. Radiation therapy is curative and should be considered for large lesions.

Subsequent Therapy

1. Treat all recurrences and any lesions with a significant palpable component by surgical excision. Microscopically controlled excision may be tissue sparing and offers a high cure rate.
2. Patients must be followed regularly for evidence of recurrence.

Pitfalls

1. The diagnosis of erythroplasia of Queyrat must be established by biopsy.
2. Too short a course of 5-FU may lead to recurrence.
3. Erythroplasia of Queyrat must be distinguished from bowenoid papulosis.

TB

68

Essential Fatty Acid Deficiency

Essential fatty acid deficiency (EFAD) is more common in premature infants and neonates owing to their increased requirements for and low body stores of the essential fatty acid linoleic acid (C18 : 2). However, both children and adults receiving prolonged parenteral nutrition, with GI malabsorption, or with chronic malnutrition are also at risk.

Initial Therapy

The best treatment is prevention. Prescribe supplements of soybean oil emulsion (Intralipid) for patients receiving prolonged intravenous nutritional supplements. Adjust the dose to ensure that at least 3% of total calories are in the form of linoleic acid.

Ancillary Therapy

1. Treat the dermatitis, if present, with an emollient ointment (e.g., hydrated petrolatum or aquaphor) b.i.d. to lubricate and restore the skin's water barrier.
2. As the diagnosis of EFAD may be difficult to distinguish from zinc deficiency, which also may co-exist with EFAD, administer supplemental zinc (zinc sulfate or other salt) 20–50 mg/day.

Alternative Therapy

Topical sunflower and safflower oils, which contain large amounts of linoleic acid, reverse the signs of EFAD in most, but not all patients. About 100 mg/kg/day of oil should be applied over the skin surface. Serum fatty acid levels must be monitored to ensure the efficacy of this approach.

Pitfalls

1. EFAD results from a variety of causes. Correction of the underlying abnormality (e.g., a GI anomaly) will result in rapid correction.
2. EFAD must be distinguished from other scaly, generalized rashes and malnutrition syndromes that may result in dermatitis. Serum fatty acids are the sine qua non of diagnosis: a C20:3 to C20:4 ratio greater than 0.4 is considered diagnostic.
3. Hypertriglyceridemia is the major complication of soybean oil emulsion infusions, particularly if the patient is receiving both oral and intravenous lipids. Acute fatty liver and pancreatitis can result, particularly in patients with pre-existing hyperlipoproteinemias. Hence, serum lipids must be monitored at regular intervals.
4. Infections at infusion sites are fairly common in patients receiving parenteral lipid emulsions.

PE

69

Exfoliative Erythroderma

Erythroderma is a clinical state that results from a variety of specific dermatologic disorders, including psoriasis, pityriasis rubra pilaris, contact dermatitis, atopic dermatitis, drug reactions, and cutaneous T-cell lymphoma, as well as underlying malignancies. Specific therapy requires the proper diagnosis. Regardless of diagnosis, however, all erythrodermas may initially be treated in a similar manner. The role of initial management is control of symptoms and relief of inflammation and erythroderma. Specific treatment must be tailored to the disease causing erythroderma.

Initial Therapy

Hospitalization is usually required, as an aggressive topical approach is too complex and demanding for home care, and elderly patients are at risk for significant medical complications, including high output cardiac failure, septicemia, hypothermia, pneumonia, and anemia. Therapy should include:

1. A warm, humid environment, and blankets to stop shivering.
2. Soaking in warm water, without soap, for 10–15 minutes, then rapidly patting the body dry with soft towels.
3. After each bath, application of a medium-potency steroid in a preservative-free ointment (e.g., Synalar ointment 0.05%; see Appendix 1).
4. Hydroxyzine 25–50 mg t.i.d. or q.i.d. for control of itch and sedation.
5. A high-protein diet with B vitamins, iron supplementation, and adequate nutrition, which are essential in this catabolic state.

Alternative Therapy

1. Antibiotics (e.g., erythromycin 250 mg q.i.d. or dicloxacillin 250 mg q.i.d.) are recommended by some, but are not generally necessary and may add to the risk of a drug reaction, which may remain a diagnostic possibility.
2. Warm saline compresses may replace soaks. Such therapy requires extensive nursing time, however, and is no more effective than soaks alone.

3. Oilated colloidal oatmeal (Aveeno) may be added to water during soaks. While not essential, such agents are soothing.

Subsequent Therapy

During initial therapy, the diagnosis of the disorder causing erythroderma must be sought. Once the diagnosis is made, specific long-term therapy can be initiated; these therapies are covered in chapters concerned with specific diseases that cause erythroderma.

Pitfalls

1. Avoid systemic steroids as initial therapy. Most patients benefit from topical therapy, and systemic steroids may cause long-term management problems in erythrodermas caused by psoriasis.
2. Carefully monitor for medical complications of erythroderma, including high-output cardiac failure, septicemia, hypothermia, anemia, and pneumonia.

BW

70

Extramammary Paget's/ Paget's Disease

Initial Therapy

1. Evaluate the patient for an underlying carcinoma of the breast (Paget's) or sweat gland, lower GU tract, or lower GI tract (extramammary Paget's). Mammary Paget's is almost always associated with an underlying carcinoma. The data on extramammary Paget's are less clear, but between 25% and 50% have an associated carcinoma. A careful lymph node evaluation is essential. Determine therapy in consultation with other appropriate surgical specialists.

2. Refer patients with Paget's disease of the breast to a general surgeon with experience in the management of breast cancer.
3. If underlying carcinoma is found in a case of extramammary Paget's referral to an appropriate surgeon (i.e., GU tract to a urologist, female genital tract to a gynecologic cancer specialist, and GI tract to a general surgeon) is indicated.
4. Extramammary Paget's, if small and not associated with underlying carcinoma, may be totally excised. Careful evaluation of the margins is essential. Some dermatologic chemosurgeons believe they can remove these lesions and spare tissue by tracing the involvement.

Alternative Therapy

Radiation therapy may be used when there is no associated underlying carcinoma, and when surgical excision is not ideal owing to the large size of the lesion or debility of the patient.

Subsequent Therapy

Careful follow-up is essential, as the recurrence rate is high following all forms of therapy. A previously occult malignancy of the GI or GU tract should be sought constantly.

Pitfalls

1. Failure to evaluate and follow up regularly for underlying malignancy.
2. All forms of therapy are associated with high recurrence and mortality rates. Therapy must be determined in consultation with appropriate surgical specialists in a Tumor Board setting.

TB

71

Flushing

Flushing can occur as an isolated disease entity owing to adrenergic hyperactivity; it can be associated with various endocrine-metabolic disorders (e.g., carcinoid tumors, pheochromocytoma, mastocytosis, hormonal insufficiency states, brain tumors) or with the use of certain drugs; and finally, it can occur as a manifestation of rosacea.

Initial Therapy

1. Adminsiter a β-blocker, such as propanalol (Inderal) 20 mg t.i.d. before meals, increasing the dose slowly as tolerated (do not use this therapy in patients with asthma, cardiac insufficiency, or possible pheochromocytoma).
2. Search for and remove dietary (gustatory flushing) or environmental etiologic agents. Spicy foods, alcohol, coffee, tea, sunlight, mushrooms, sulfite preservatives in fresh fruits and vegetables, cyclamates, and monosodium glutamate (Accent) should be avoided if a relationship can be shown. Exposure to certain solvent vapors (e.g., trichlorethylene) also can induce flushing.
3. Look for drug-related causes: antabuse or metronidazole (Flagyl) with alcohol, nicotinic acid, chlorpropamide, griseofulvin, and cephalosporins are also occasional offenders.
4. Perform a diagnostic work-up on all patients with flushing for a possible underlying cause: measure urinary 5-HIAA, blood histamine, plasma catecholamines, and urinary vasoactive intestinal peptide (VIP). Evaluate patients with associated diarrhea for mastocytosis (CBC, upper GI series with small bowel follow-through, liver-spleen scan, and bone marrow examination). A CT scan is indicated to rule out a brain tumor in patients with associated migraine headaches and/or orthostatic hypotension.

Alternative Therapy

1. For flushing with sweating, the anticholinergic agent propantheline bromide 15 mg t.i.d. can be used with or without a β-blocker.
2. For patients unresponsive to propanolol and/or propantheline, antihis-

tamines (both H_1 and H_2 blockers; chlorpheniramine maleate 8–16 mg/day, and cimetidine 100 mg t.i.d.).

3. Patients unresponsive to both adrenergic and histamine blockades next should be administered inhibitors of eicosanoid synthesis (i.e., indomethacin 25 mg b.i.d., increasing to 50 mg b.i.d., or aspirin 6–8 tablets/day).

4. The next alternative is the antiserotonin agent cyproheptidine (Periactin initially 4 mg b.i.d.) and/or chlorpromazine 25 mg t.i.d., the latter for its antibradykinin activity.

5. Clonidine 25-75 μg b.i.d. or diethylstilbestrol 2 mg/day may be useful for patients with menopausal flushing. However, β-blockers are also effective here.

6. Finally, systemic steroids (e.g., oral triamcinalone acetate (Kenalog) 40–80 mg/day or prednisone 15 mg/day) can be used for temporary relief or for more long-term relief, if necessary.

Ancillary Therapy

1. For gustatory flushing, cheeses, chocolate, lemons, and highly spiced foods such as chili peppers (capsaicin is the offending ingredient) are to be avoided.

2. For auriculotemporal sweating associated with flushing, a cream containing scopolamine 3% or atropine 0.5% can be applied q.a.m. or immediately before eating.

3. Cool external temperatures at times of eating often will reduce the severity and frequency of flushing episodes.

4. Sunscreens containing both UVB and UVA blocking ingredients can alleviate sun-induced episodes.

5. Tetracycline 250–750 mg/day, when given for associated rosacea (see Ch. 154), may decrease the severity and frequency of flushing episodes. Moreover, tetracycline also improves and prevents progression of telangiectasias.

6. Pyridoxine 50 mg/day will prevent Chinese restaurant syndrome (see above).

Pitfalls

1. Patients with drug-related flushing episodes should receive treatment aimed at the specific drug interaction responsible for flushing rather than nonspecific therapy (see Shelley WB, Shelley ED: Advanced Dermatologic Therapy, WB Saunders, Philadelphia, 1987, p. 196–201, for a list of various drug interactions and therapies).

2. The failure to search for an underlying cause of flushing (see above).
3. The side effects of β-blockers are discussed in Chapter 65.
4. The side effects of systemic steroid therapy are discussed in Appendix 5.
5. All of the other drugs suggested above can produce distinctive adverse reactions or side effects. Consult the PDR before prescribing these agents.

PE

72

Folliculitis

Folliculitis is almost always caused by penicillin-resistant strains of *S. aureus*. Gram-negative forms occur, usually on the face, in the setting of chronic, broad-spectrum antibiotic therapy of acne vulgaris. Since inflammation is limited to the hair follicle, classic signs of infection (dolor, calor, rubor, and tumor) may be absent, making differentiation from milaria, papulovesicular viral exanthems, and acneiform eruptions difficult. Samples should be obtained for Gram stain and/or culture.

Initial Therapy

1. Either oral dicloxacillin 250 mg q.i.d. or oral erythromycin (in penicillin-allergic individuals) 250 mg q.i.d. for 10 days.
2. Alternate initial therapy for methicillin- or erythromycin-resistant strains, which are increasing in frequency: Trimethoprim-sulfamethoxazole (either Septra DS or Bactrim DS) 1 tablet b.i.d. or ciprofloxacin 500 mg b.i.d. (the latter should be taken on an empty stomach, and is contraindicated in children).
3. Gram-negative folliculitis: After obtaining pretreatment laboratory studies, a single course of isotretinoin 40 mg b.i.d. for 16 weeks usually is curative. Note: Cultures should be repeated 1–3 weeks after initiation of therapy, and at the end of treatment course.

Ancillary Therapy

1. Instruct the patient to shower daily with either chlorhexidine (Hibiclens) or povidone-iodine (Betadine). Close contacts of patients also should use antiseptic cleansers over the same time period to avoid transmittance within the family and/or recurrences.

2. The skin of the buttocks is particularly susceptible to recurrent episodes of folliculitis. The frequency of such episodes can be decreased with the wearing of loose-fitting cotton underwear, loose-fitting trousers, frequent applications of an astringent powder (e.g., Zeasorb) to shorts, and/or daily applications of an astringent solution (e.g., aluminum chloride (Xerac-AC)).

Pitfalls

1. Persistent nasal carriage may occur in partially treated cases. Such patients should be treated with either dicloxacillin (cephalexin for penicillin-allergic individuals) 250 mg q.i.d. plus rifampicin 300 mg b.i.d. for 7 days, or clindamycin alone 150 mg q.i.d. for 7 days.

2. Relapses are common owing to persistent nasal carriage, transmission between family members, inadequate length of treatment, emergence of methicillin-resistant strains (recurrent lesions should be recultured), and rarely, an underlying immunologic abnormality. When relapses occur, a prolonged course of therapy (i.e., 3 months) with low-dose clindamycin 150 mg/day will result in permanent clearing in about 80% of patients.

3. The side effects of systemic retinoid treatment are described in Appendix 6.

4. Systemic clindamycin therapy can cause severe colitis.

5. Rifampicin causes the urine to develop an orange tinge.

PE

73

Fox-Fordyce Disease

Apocrine Miliaria

Recalcitrant, recurrent itching in the axillary, genital, and areolar areas over many years is the primary symptom. Fox-Fordyce disease occurs almost solely in women, and may flare in relation to menses.

Initial Therapy

High-potency topical fluorinated steroids (see Appendix 1) may be given for 2 weeks initially (switch to low-potency steroids for the axillae and groin thereafter). High-potency preparations can be used for longer periods on the areolae, but all patients should be switched to lower-potency preparations as soon as relief is achieved.

Alternative Therapy

1. Estrogen-dominant OCPs (e.g., Enovid-E) will control symptoms in most women not helped by topical steroids.
2. Diethylstilbestrol (1.25–5 mg/day) can be given to post menopausal women not responding to OCPs.
3. Application of retinoic acid (Retin-A) 0.05% cream q.h.s. may be helpful in some patients.
4. Some patients may benefit from surgical excision of localized, recalcitrant areas of pruritus.

Subsequent Therapy

1. Switch from potent topical steroids to medium- or low-potency preparations (e.g., desonide) as soon as relief occurs.
2. Likewise, patients taking diethylstilbestrol should be switched to estrogen-dominant OCPs to reduce risks of high-dose estrogen therapy.
3. Groin and axillary symptoms in some patients are relieved by applications of one or more of the following: aluminum chloride 6%, (Xerac-AC) aluminum chloride 20% (Drysol), and/or an astringent powder (Zeasorb).

Pitfalls

1. The risk of skin atrophy from topical steroids is especially great in occluded areas, such as the axillae and groin.
2. Thromboembolic complications are the main complication of estrogens, although migraine headaches and hypertension also occur with increased frequency.

PE

74

Furuncles and Carbuncles

Boils

Furunculosis is almost always caused by invasive, penicillin-resistant strains of *S. aureus*, and requires vigorous antibiotic therapy.

Initial Therapy

1. Incise and drain fluctuant lesions and take a sample for culture and sensitivity. Antibiotic coverage is not usually helpful as the sole therapy, but is useful for eliminating skin and mucosal carriage, as well as subsequent recurrences.
2. Dicloxacillin 250–500 mg q.i.d. for 2 weeks is of benefit.
3. Treat the anterior nares with a topical antibiotic ointment such as bacitracin, neosporin, or mupirocin (Bactroban) q.d. applied with a cotton-tipped applicator. Note: The efficacy of topical antibiotics for nasal carriage has been questionable. For systemic therapy, see Ancillary Therapy, below.

Alternative Therapy

1. Penicillin-allergic individuals should be treated with either erythromycin 1 g/day or cephalexin 250–500 mg q.i.d. for 2 weeks.
2. Methicillin-resistant strains can be treated with trimethoprim-

sulfamethoxazole (Septra DS or Bactrim DS) 1 tablet b.i.d., clindamycin (Cleocin) 150 mg q.i.d., or ciprofloxacin 500 mg b.i.d. on an empty stomach.

Ancillary Therapy

1. Family members can harbor organisms, resulting in recurrent infections within the family. All family members should treat external nares with one of the topical antibiotics listed above, and shower daily with chlorhexidine (Hibiclens) or povidone-iodine (Betadine) for at least 5 days.
2. The skin of the buttocks is particularly susceptible to recurrent episodes of folliculitis and/or furunculosis. The frequency of such episodes can be decreased with the wearing of loose-fitting cotton underwear, loose-fitting trousers, frequent applications of an astringent powder (e.g., Zeasorb) to shorts, and/or daily applications of an astringent solution (e.g., aluminum chloride (Xerac-AC)).
3. Persistent nasal carriage that is unresponsive to topical therapy should be treated with either dicloxacillin (cephalexin for penicillin-allergic individuals) 250 mg q.i.d. for 10–14 days plus refampicin 300 mg b.i.d. for 7 days or clindamycin alone 150 mg q.i.d. for 7 days.

Pitfalls

1. Relapses are common, owing to persistent nasal carriage, transmission between family members, inadequate length of treatment, emergence of methicillin-resistant strains (reculture recurrent lesions), and rarely, an underlying immunologic abnormality. When relapses occur, a prolonged course of low-dose clindamycin 150 mg/day for 3 months produces permanent clearing in about 80% of patients.
2. If treatment for persistent nasal carriage is unsuccessful, evaluate patients with recurrent episodes of furunculosis for an immunologic deficiency or an abnormality of phagocyte function.
3. Acne cysts and hidradenitis suppurativa can be confused with furuncles.
4. Systemic clindamycin therapy can cause severe colitis.
5. Rifampicin causes the urine to develop an orange tinge.

PE

75

Geographic Tongue

Annulus Migrans

Initial Therapy

Vitamin A acid (Retin-A) 0.025% gel may be applied to the tongue b.i.d.

TB

76

Gianotti–Crosti Syndrome

Although classically associated with hepatitis B infections, acute papular acrodermatitis or Gianotti-Crosti syndrome (GCS) can follow *Mycoplasma* or several types of viral infections. The presence of petechiae in the rash, however, usually indicates hepatitis B as the cause.

Initial Therapy

1. The therapy for *Mycoplasma*-associated eruptions is erythromycin 30–50 mg/kg/day, divided in four doses for at least 3 weeks. In other cases the rash is self-limited, typically resolving in 21 days.
2. Minimum work-up includes CBC, liver enzymes, acute and convalescent serologic tests for Epstein–Barr virus, and hepatitis A and B antigens and antibodies. Cold agglutinins and a positive chest x-ray are the most useful indicators of *Mycoplasma* infection.

Ancillary Therapy

1. For nonspecific, symptomatic therapy of fever and pruritus associated with viral exanthems, see Chapter 183.
2. GCS can spread in epidemics, both within families and in schools. Serologic tests for hepatitis should be obtained from all family members of patients with GCS, and antibody-negative relatives should receive active hepatitis immunization.
3. Topical steroids may exacerbate the rash in GCS.

Pitfalls

Acute hepatitis, in GCS, although usually asymptomatic, may progress to chronic active hepatitis. Therefore, patients and infected family members should have repeat LFTs 4–8 weeks after resolution of the disease.

PE

77

Gonorrhea and Disseminated Gonococcemia

Gonococcal infection may remain localized to one or several mucosal surfaces or may become blood borne, causing a characteristic dermatitis-arthritis syndrome. Neonatal gonorrhea, gonococcal meningitis, and gonococcal endocarditis are not discussed. Penicillin-resistant (PPNG) strains are common in some geographic areas and therapy must be directed accordingly.

Initial Therapy

1. For local mucosal disease (urethral, cervical, rectal, pharyngeal): Intramuscular ceftriaxone 250 mg in one dose. For children under 45 kg, 125 mg in one dose (adequate for PPNG strains).

2. For disseminated gonococcemia (with or without arthritis): Intravenous ceftriaxone 1 g/day for 7 days (adequate for PPNG strains).
3. Evaluate the patient for other STDs.
4. Treat the patient for coexistent chlamydial urethritis with doxycycline 100 mg b.i.d. or tetracycline or erythromycin 500 mg q.i.d. for 7 days.

Alternative Therapy

1. For urethral or cervical disease: Oral amoxicillin 3 g plus oral probenecid 1 g in one dose. For PPNG strains: Intramuscular spectinomycin 2 g in one dose.
2. For rectal disease: Intramuscular procaine penicillin G 4.8×10^6 U plus oral probenecid 1 g in one dose. For PPNG strains: Intramuscular spectinomycin 2 g.
3. For pharyngeal disease: Intramuscular procaine penicillin G 4.8×10^6 U plus oral probenecid 1 g in one dose. For PPNG strains: trimethoprim 80 mg-sulfamethoxazole 400 mg, 9 tablets/day in one dose for 5 days.
4. For bacteremia (and arthritis): Intravenous penicillin G 10×10^6 U/day for 3 days followed by oral amoxicillin 500 mg q.i.d. for 4 days.

Subsequent Therapy

For all patients, but especially those harboring PPNG strains, obtain repeat cultures of affected sites after 4–7 days to document cure.

Pitfalls

1. Due to the rise in PPNG strains in the United States, be constantly aware of whether these strains exist in your community. If they do exist, initial therapy should cover these strains. Perform cultures on all suspected gonorrhea cases and report positive results to the appropriate community agency.
2. Failure to look for and treat other STDs in patients with gonorrhea is a common error. Do a complete examination.

TB

78

Granuloma Annulare

The effectiveness of therapy of granuloma annulare (GA) may be difficult to gauge because spontaneous resolution of individual lesions or the entire disease process is common. Performance of a skin biopsy alone is often enough to trigger spontaneous resolution.

Initial Therapy

1. Prescribe a superpotent topical steroid to be applied to lesions in a thin film b.i.d. Although GA is a dermal inflammatory disease, a substantial percentage of lesions will respond to this therapy within 2–4 weeks.
2. *Alternative initial therapy:* Apply squares of flurandrenolide-impregnated tape (Cordran) to lesions for 12–24 hours, or prescribe an intermediate-potency topical steroid (e.g., triamcinolone acetonide (Kenalog) 0.1% cream) under plastic wrap or plastic glove occlusion overnight.

Alternative Therapy

1. Inject intralesional steroids (triamcinolone acetonide 10 mg/cc) diluted 1 : 3 with normal saline using a 30-gauge needle. Injections can be repeated very 3–4 weeks. *Note:* Be careful not to inject the steroid solution too superficially to avoid cutaneous atrophy. Aim for the middle-to-deep part of the lesion.
2. Several uncontrolled studies claim success with platelet-disaggregating agents. A regimen of dipyridamole (Persantin) 50 mg t.i.d. and aspirin 165 mg (1/2 tablet) b.i.d. may be useful for generalized or widespread GA.
3. Potassium iodide 5 drops of the supersaturated solution (SSKI) t.i.d. increasing to 10 drops t.i.d., taken in a glass of water or citrus fruit juice, is effective in a significant proportion of patients, although lesions recur following cessation of therapy.
4. Pentoxyphylline (Trental) 400 mg/day, increasing to t.i.d., has been reported to induce remissions in over 50% of patients with generalized GA within 3–4 weeks.
5. Although there are reports of dapsone, systemic corticosteroids, and alkylating agents (chlorambucil) inducing remissions in GA, their administration is rarely, if ever, justified.

Pitfalls

1. There may be an association between generalized, extensive GA and diabetes mellitus. If not recently evaluated, patients with GA should have a routine fasting blood sugar or glucose tolerance test.
2. The pitfalls of topical and systemic corticosteroids are described in Appendices 3 and 5.
3. The pitfalls of oral potassium iodide therapy are described in Chapter 162, Sporotrichosis.
4. The pitfalls of platelet-disaggregating agents and pentoxiphylline include increased risk of gastrointestinal bleeding, especially if both types of agents are used concurrently, or in patients with peptic ulcer disease or on oral anticoagulants. In patients with concurrent coronary artery disease, angina, arrhythmias, and hypotension have been reported. Dizziness, headache, and other nervous system symptoms occur occasionally, and miscellaneous gastrointestinal side effects, such as nausea and bloating, may occur.

79

Granuloma Faciale

All modes of therapy for granuloma faciale may be followed by recurrence.

Initial Therapy

1. Dapsone 100 mg/day often leads to resolution of existing lesions. Occasionally doses up to 200 mg/day may be required.
2. Phenylbutazone 100 mg t.i.d. may also be beneficial.

Alternative Therapy

1. Intralesional injections of triamcinolone acetonide (Kenalog) 5 mg/cc are occasionally of benefit.
2. Chloroquine 500 mg/day has been reported as beneficial. Due to the risk of retinopathy, exercise care in the use of this agent for this disease.
3. Topical PUVA for 10 weeks reportedly cleared one patient's disease.
4. Clofazamine 300 mg/day was also beneficial in a single case.

Subsequent Therapy

1. Patients failing to respond to the above therapies may be treated surgically: dermabrasion, excision, electrodesiccation, cryotherapy, and laser have all been reported as effective.
2. Patients responding to dapsone may require constant treatment, although the maintenance dose may be much lower, 25–50 mg/day.

Pitfalls

1. Recurrence is common, so beware of overzealous scarring therapy. Patient informed consent is vital.
2. Dapsone therapy may lead to anemia. A baseline CBC, G6PD, and LFTs are required. Regular monitoring of the CBC and LFTs during therapy is advised. For pitfalls of dapsone therapy, see Chapter 84, Hansen's disease.

TB

80

Granuloma Fissuratum

Granuloma fissuratum is related to chronic friction from an artificial substance at the site of a fold. The two most common locations are the mouth (from dentures) and the retroauricular sulcus (from eyeglasses).

Initial Therapy

Refer the patient to an optician for refitting of the eyeglass frames or to the dentist for refitting of the dentures.

Pitfall

A basal cell carcinoma behind the ear may be clinically very similar, and a biopsy may be necessary to establish the correct diagnosis.

TB

81

Granuloma Inguinale

Initial Therapy

Oral tetracycline 500 mg q.i.d. Treatment must be continued for at least 3 weeks, or until the patient is clear of disease. Clinical response should be noted in 7 days.

Alternative Therapy

1. Trimethoprim 160 mg-sulfamethoxazole 800 mg b.i.d., or
2. Minocycline 100 mg b.i.d.

Subsequent Therapy

For cases failing the above therapies try:

1. Erythromycin or lincomycin 500 mg q.i.d., or
2. Chloramphenicol 500 mg t.i.d., or
3. Intramuscular streptomycin 1 g b.i.d., or
4. Intramuscular gentamicin 1 mg/kg b.i.d.

Pitfalls

1. Due to its rarity in most western countries, this diagnosis is frequently overlooked. Touch preparations and/or biopsies are required to establish the diagnosis and to rule out a squamous cell carcinoma in some cases.
2. Early discontinuation of treatment leads to more frequent relapse.
3. Although chloramphenicol and gentamicin are highly effective, restrict their use to patients failing to respond to other safer agents.
4. Evaluate the patient for other STDs.

TB

82

Hailey—Hailey Disease

Hailey-Hailey disease (HHD), also called *benign familial pemphigus*, is an autosomal-dominant disorder. A characteristic histology differentiates HHD from the seborrheic variant of Darier's disease (keratosis follicularis). Since no specific therapy is available, management can be difficult. HHD most frequently involves interriginous areas, where exacerbations are triggered by heat, sweating, friction, and/or secondary infections. Hence, therapy is aimed at minimizing all of these provocative factors.

Initial Therapy

1. Prescribe applications of an astringent, either aluminum chloride 6% in a roll-on preparation (Xerac-AC) b.i.d., or for more severe cases, aluminum chloride 20% solution (Drysol) q.d.
2. Immediately after application of astringent, a topical antibiotic (e.g., either erythromycin 2% solution (e.g., T/Stat or Eryderm) or clindamycin 1% solution (Cleocin-T)) should be applied.
3. After both astringent and topical antibiotic applications, an absorbent powder (e.g., Zeasorb) should be applied. *Note:* Cornstarch is a nutritious substrate for microbes; hence, it has no place in modern topical therapy.
4. If secondary infection is already apparent and/or if cultures reveal the presence of pathogenic bacteria (usually *S. aureus*), then administer appropriate oral antibiotics (e.g., dicloxacillin 250 mg q.i.d. for 14 days, or for penicillin-allergic patients, erythromycin 250 mg q.i.d. × 14 days).
5. Showers or baths with antibacterial cleansers (e.g., clorhexidine (Hibiclens) or povidone-iodine (Betadine)).

Alternative Therapy

Dapsone 25 mg b.i.d., increasing to a total dosage of 200–300 mg/day, may be useful for patients with disease not controlled with the topical program outlined above.

Subsequent Therapy

1. Gauge the intensity of therapy against disease severity and the number of involved sites.
2. Seasonal exacerbations occur, not due to ultraviolet light (as in Darier's disease), but rather to increased heat, sweating, friction, and bacterial colonization in warmer months. Hence, therapy can often be adjusted on a seasonal basis.
3. Severely involved patients may benefit from surgical excision of chronically affected, intertriginous areas.

Pitfalls

1. The increasing incidence of erythromycin-resistant strains of staphylococci means that erythromycin should be used only when sensitivities indicate its use, and not as prophylactic therapy. In fact, prophylactic antibiotics should be avoided to minimize the emergence of resistant strains.
2. Resident microflora also can develop in situ resistance to *topical* antibiotics. Hence, if long-term topical antibiotics are employed, clindamycin (Cleocin-T) and erythromycin should be alternated at about 3-month intervals.
3. Although HHD is classified with the disorders of cornification, such as Darier's disease and the ichthyoses, it is not helped and even may be exacerbated by the currently available systemic retinoids acitretin, etretinate (Tegison), or isotretinoin (Accutane).
4. Dapsone can produce acute hemolysis in patients who are G6PD deficient; therefore, blood serum for enzyme activity must be obtained prior to initiating therapy. For other types of toxicity associated with dapsone therapy, see Chapter 43, Dermatitis Herpetiformis.

PE

83

Hand Eczema

Hand eczema can range from an acute, extremely pruritic or painful eruption, characterized by minute, "tapioca" vesicles (dyshidrotic eczema, pompholyx), to the chronic hand eczema commonly seen in housewives or those in other at-risk occupations (e.g., bartenders).

DYSHIDROTIC (ACUTE) HAND ECZEMA

Initial Therapy

1. A single intramuscular injection of triamcinolone acetonide (Kenalog) 40–80 mg is extremely helpful for acute relief, but should be reserved for severely affected patients.
2. Antihistamines are administered both to decrease pruritus and for their central, sedating activity. Prescribe doxepin 25 mg q.p.m. initially, with the dose increased to 50–75 mg as patients become accustomed to the soporific effects of this agent.

Ancillary Therapy

1. Domeboro soaks (1 tablet or packet/pt cool tap water) for 15 minutes b.i.d. will relieve itching and reduce likelihood of secondary infection.
2. A superpotent or high-potency topical fluorinated steroid cream (see Appendix 1) should be applied q.d. or b.i.d. after soaks.

Alternative Therapy

1. Photochemotherapy (PUVA), administered with a hand and foot unit, can be very effective, but this modality takes several weeks to produce remission, and is available only in selected dermatologists' offices or tertiary facilities.
2. A high-potency topical, fluorinated steroid (see Appendix 1) can be applied under occlusion (plastic-wrap or vinyl gloves) overnight. This is an effective alternative in patients who should not receive systemic steroids.
3. Soaks in a tar emulsion (Balnetar or Zetar), followed by UVB phototherapy are effective, but again require a specialized facility or light source.

Subsequent Therapy

Many patients with dyshidrotic eczema are atopics and require counseling about avoidance of hot water and harsh soaps. Moreover, they should be encouraged to wear rubber gloves for protection, use a mild, oilated or glycerated soap, and apply a hand cream or ointment (e.g., Aquaphor (Eucerin) or hydrated petroleum (Vaseline)) after each hand-washing.

CHRONIC HAND ECZEMA

Initial Therapy

Prescribe a high-potency or superpotent topical, fluorinated steroid *ointment* (see Appendix 1) to be applied q.d. or b.i.d. Alternatively, a medium-potency steroid cream can be applied under occlusion (using plastic wrap or vinyl gloves) q.h.s., overnight.

Ancillary Therapy

1. Almost all patients with chronic hand eczema are atopics, and suffer disease exacerbations from excessive exposure to hot water and harsh detergents. Hence, use of cool water, mild soaps, adequate protection, and an emollient hand cream is critical to prevent relapses in these patients.
2. Antihistamines (e.g., hydroxyzine 25 mg q.i.d.) may be helpful for the initial control of pruritus.
3. Patients with recalcitrant and/or recurrent disease may benefit from concurrent therapy with a cosmetically acceptable tar preparation (e.g., Fototar cream) applied q.d. concurrent with or separately from topical steroids. Use of tar makes the dermatitis less dependent on steroids and hence, less likely to relapse, as well as minimizes the possible side effects from topical steroids.

Alternative Therapy

1. Some patients with severe or persistent hand eczema may benefit from a short course of systemic steroids (e.g., intramuscular triamcinolone acetonide 40–60 mg).
2. Patients with severe, recalcitrant hand eczema may be candidates for topical PUVA or tar–UVB phototherapy (see above).

Pitfalls

1. Check patients with acute dyshidrotic eczema for inflammatory tinea pedis or active stasis dermatitis (SD). SD reactions (auto sensitization) from these two conditions can mimic dyshidrotic eczema. Occasionally, an allergic contact dermatitis, restricted to the palms, will mimic chronic hand eczema. In suspected allergic contact dermatitis, patch testing may be required to detect the responsible allergen.

2. Both acute and chronic hand eczema can become secondarily infected, usually with *S. aureus*. The presence of honey-colored crusts should alert one to this complication, which can exacerbate the pruritus in these patients. Dicloxacillin or erythromycin 250 mg q.i.d. for 7–10 days is almost always curative.

3. If effective topical therapy is not administered simultaneously with intramuscular steroids, relapse is the rule. Moreover, the effectiveness of intermittent, systemic steroid therapy tends to produce dependency, thereby increasing potential complications of systemic corticosteroid therapy (see Appendix 5).

4. Both acute and chronic hand eczema tend to relapse and/or persist for years. A preventive program, consisting of antihistamines, protective gloves, cool water washing, mild soaps, and frequent application of emollients is required for long-term control.

5. Although tachyphylaxis occurs within a few days, antihistamines are sedating, and patients must be warned about operating motor vehicles or other tasks requiring fine motor skills during initial therapy.

6. Neither UVB phototherapy nor PUVA is curative for hand eczema. Long-term therapy is required to maintain remissions.

7. Nonsteroidal anti-inflammatory agents may cause a hand dermatitis with dyshidrosiform features, but with more dorsal than palmar involvement.

PE

84

Hansen's Disease and Reactional States

Leprosy

Optimal therapeutic regimens for Hansen's disease (HD) have not been established by controlled trials. Therapy is determined primarily by the bacillary load (i.e., multibacillary vs. paucibacillary). Multibacillary patients include all lepromatous and almost all borderline patients (except those near the tuberculoid pole). Paucibacillary patients are those with indeterminate, pure tuberculoid, and borderline tuberculoid leprosy, in which organisms are absent or extremely hard to find by smears and biopsy. Other factors important in determining therapy are the availability of medications, the likelihood of dapsone resistance, and the compliance of the patient. The World Health Organization (WHO) has recommended limited or fixed courses of therapy with multiple agents to enhance compliance, reduce cost, and manage dapsone resistance. Because of the unique features of this disease and the lack of experience of most practitioners in the management of HD, early in the course of evaluation, an experienced leprologist should evaluate the patient and guide therapy. A determination of dapsone sensitivity may be made by culture in mouse foot pad, and should be considered in all multibacillary patients prior to any treatment. The management of reactional states is discussed at the end of this section.

Initial Therapy

DAPSONE-SENSITIVE BACILLI

1. Paucibacillary patients: dapsone 100 mg/day plus rifampin 600 mg q.d., unsupervised; or rifampin 600 mg once monthly, supervised for 6 months.
2. Multibacillary patients: dapsone 100 mg/day plus rifampin 600 mg q.d.,

unsupervised; or rifampin 600 mg once monthly, supervised for 3 years. Additionally, consider ethionamide 250–500 mg/day or clofazamine 50–100 mg/day, especially if there is a possibility of dapsone resistance.

DAPSONE-RESISTANT BACILLI

1. Paucibacillary patients: clofazamine 50–100 mg/day plus rifampin 600 mg/day or 600 mg once monthly, supervised for 6 months.
2. Multibacillary patients: clofazamine 50–100 mg/day plus rifampin 600 mg/day or 600 mg once monthly, supervised for 3 years. Ethionamide or prothionamide 250–500 mg/day may be added, and is required if the patient refuses to take clofazamine.

Subsequent Therapy

Drug therapy is continued until an inactive status (negative scrapings for 1 year, negative biopsy, and no evidence of disease activity, such as reaction_or progressive neurologic deficit) is achieved.

DAPSONE-SENSITIVE BACILLI

1. Paucibacillary patients: Dapsone 100 mg/day for 3–5 years.
2. Multibacillary patients: Dapsone 100 mg/day for 10 years–life.

DAPSONE-RESISTANT BACILLI

1. Paucibacillary patients: Clofazamine 50–100 mg/day for 3–5 years.
2. Multibacillary patients: Clofazamine 50–100 mg/day for 10 years–life.
3. For patients refusing clofazamine, rifampin 600 mg/day plus ethionamide or prothionamide 250–500 mg/day for the periods recommended above.

Pitfalls

1. The initial evaluation by a leprologist should be performed before any effective therapy has been given.
2. A strong psychological support program is required when initially diagnosing HD. Patients may feel very stigmatized, and depression to the point of suicide is possible.
3. Rifampin and ethionamide-prothionamide together or alone may cause hepatotoxicity. If significant abnormalities of the LFTs occur (more than doubling of the SGOT or SGPT) both drugs should be stopped. When LFTs return to normal the rifampin may be reinstituted. Rifampin may rarely cause thrombocytopenia. Patients taking rifampin will note a reddish-

acyclovir resistance may rarely appear in immunosuppressed, especially HIV-infected, persons. Systemic and neonatal HSV infections are not discussed.

Initial Therapy

1. For primary orofacial HSV and primary genital HSV patients, immunocompromised patients, and eczema herpeticum patients:
   a. Oral acyclovir 200 mg 5×/day while awake (about every 4 hours). For hospitalized patients with intravenous lines, or for those with HSV infection requiring hospitalization: Intravenous acyclovir 5 mg/kg t.i.d. (adjusted for renal function). Therapy is continued for 5 days. If lesions are still present after this time continue acyclovir therapy another 5 days.
   b. Soaks or sitz baths to dry the blisters or remove crusts may be adjunctively beneficial.
   c. Culture for coexistent bacterial superinfection (usually *S. aureus*) and treat appropriately.
   d. For eczema herpeticum: Treat the atopic dermatitis.
   e. For genital HSV: Evaluate for other STDs.
   f. For the immunosuppressed, topical acyclovir ointment 4–5×/day may accelerate healing.
2. Recurrent orofacial HSV responds to drying preparations (e.g., benzoyl peroxide gel) b.i.d. Oral and topical acyclovir do not significantly shorten the course in most patients once lesions are present.
3. Recurrent genital HSV episodes may be slightly shortened by oral acyclovir 200 mg q.4h. while awake (5×/day) for 5 days. It must be begun at the earliest prodrome and be patient initiated. Topical acyclovir ointment is of almost no benefit in this setting.

Alternative Therapy

1. For the treatment of acute episodes, there is no readily available effective treatment other than acyclovir.

Subsequent Therapy

1. For primary and recurrent orofacial HSV in nonimmunosuppressed patients:
   a. Lesions are likely to recur and patients need to be so advised.
   b. Patients should avoid triggers (especially intense sun exposure), and

should use a sunscreen on the face and a lip balm containing a sunscreen.

    c. Sun exposure-triggered recurrent orofacial HSV may be suppressed by acyclovir 400 mg b.i.d. for 3 days prior to exposure and continued through the time of exposure. This is good for trips to the tropics and before skiing.

    d. Orolabial HSV followed by erythema multiforme is an indication for oral acyclovir suppression (400 mg b.i.d. or 200 mg t.i.d.). Therapy may be continued for up to 1 year, then after a drug "holiday" and re-evaluation, may be reinstituted.

    e. Patients undergoing lip peels, dermabrasion, or extensive dental work, which may trigger their HSV, should be given full doses of acyclovir orally (200 mg q.4h.) for 2 days prior to the surgical procedure and until the wound is healed.

2. For primary and recurrent genital HSV nonimmunosuppressed patients:

    a. Recurrence is common and patients should be so advised.

    b. Patients education is essential. When active lesions are present patients must use condoms or abstain from sexual relations involving contact of the lesion(s) with their sexual partner. Men and women with recurrent buttock lesions may shed virus from the urethra/cervix while buttocks lesions are active, and should be considered infectious. HSV may be transmitted from asymptomatic persons before lesions appear. Women may shed asymptomatically from the cervix.

    c. For frequent recurrences (more than 6–12/year) begin chronic acyclovir 400 mg b.i.d. or 200 mg t.i.d. Taper the dose to the minimal suppressive dose (usually between 1 and 4 tablets/day).

3. For immunosuppressed patients (with orofacial or genital HSV), because protracted infections may occur, oral acyclovir suppression (400 mg b.i.d.) is indicated, no matter how infrequent the outbreaks.

4. For eczema herpeticum patients:

    a. Recurrences are unusual, therefore, chronic suppression is unnecessary. Patient education, a high index of suspicion, and rapid diagnosis and institution of treatment are the keys to preventing subsequent episodes.

    b. Chronic therapy for the associated atopic dermatitis is essential.

Pitfalls

1. Failure to adjust the acyclovir dose for decreased renal function can lead to side effects, especially when high-dose intravenous acyclovir is given. (Monitor renal function during intravenous acyclovir therapy and ensure adequate hydration to prevent renal impairment.)

2. Genital ulcers are difficult to diagnose. HSV II is the most common cause of genital ulcer disease in the United States, and accurate, confirmed diagnosis is essential. Do not tell the patient they have herpes unless it is confirmed by culture or fluorescent antibody or Tzanck smear. Serologic testing is in general not useful except in the primary disease with acute and convalescent titers. The results of serologic testing are usually not available for days, and are only retrospectively of benefit in the rare case.
3. Be alert for the genital ulcer containing multiple pathogens and evaluate patients with genital HSV for other STDs.
4. Rarely acylovir-resistant mutants of HSV may cause chronic genital or oral ulcers in immunosuppressed (usually HIV-infected) patients.

TB

88

Herpes Zoster

Shingles

The management of herpes zoster includes the treatment of the acute eruption and therapy for herpetic neuralgia and postherpetic neuralgia.

ACUTE MANAGEMENT OF HERPES ZOSTER

The management of herpes zoster is dependent upon the *age of the patient*, the *location* of the eruption, the *immune competence* of the patient, and the presence of *coexistent diseases* contraindicating steroid usage (e.g., active tuberculosis, diabetes mellitus, hypertension and peptic ulcer disease).

Initial Therapy

GENERAL MEASURES FOR ALL PATIENTS

1. For blistering lesions, Burow's compresses 1 : 20 up to q.i.d. will speed drying of the lesions and removal of the crusts.

2. Silver sulfadiazine (Silvadene) cream may be applied b.i.d. to q.i.d. to prevent secondary bacterial infection and to reduce discomfort.
3. Refer all patients with ophthalmic (V1) zoster (lesions around the eye or on the nose) to an ophthalmologist within 24 hours.
4. Advise the patient to avoid contact with immunosuppressed persons and persons who have not had varicella (chicken pox) until all lesions are crusted.
5. Perform a cursory review of symptoms for previously undetected malignancy. No additional laboratory tests beyond those suggested by the physical examination and review of symptoms are required.

PATIENTS UNDER 50 YEARS, IMMUNOCOMPETENT

Most immunocompetent younger patients are not benefitted by antiviral therapy. Infections of the ophthalmic branch (V1) of the trigeminal nerve and the Ramsey-Hunt syndrome (facial palsy and herpes zoster oticus) may be exceptions, where oral acyclovir 800 mg 5×/day may reduce morbidity. (Correct the dosage for renal function.)

PATIENTS OVER 50 YEARS, IMMUNOCOMPETENT

1. Patients over 50 are at higher risk for postherpetic neuralgia. Although brought into question by recent studies, the currently accepted therapy to reduce the likelihood of postherpetic neuralgia is 3 weeks of oral prednisone 60 mg in a single morning dose with food for the first week, 40 mg for the second week, and 20 mg for the third week. Patients must be evaluated for contraindications to systemic corticosteroids.
2. In this population oral acyclovir may speed healing and reduce acute pain. If given, use full doses (800 mg p.o. 5×/day). (Correct the dosage for renal function.)

IMMUNOSUPPRESSED PATIENTS

Except for those who are severely immunosuppressed, the risk of cutaneous dissemination is low and visceral dissemination is uncommon. These patients do tend to have a more prolonged course, more pain, more extradermatomal lesions, and more scarring. Not all immunosuppressed patients require acyclovir therapy, but those who are not treated should be followed carefully for dissemination.

1. Administer oral acyclovir 800 mg 5×/day to moderately immunosuppressed patients without evidence of visceral dissemination. (Correct the dosage for renal function.)

2. In severely immunosuppressed patients who are at high risk for or who have dissemination only intravenous acyclovir (10 mg/kg or 500 mg/m^2 body surface area q.8h.) can be guaranteed to reach adequate tissue levels to prevent or treat disseminated zoster. (Correct the dosage for renal function.)
3. Isolate hospitalized patients from other immunosuppressed persons. Staff without a prior history of varicella should not enter their rooms.
4. The risk of dissemination is enhanced by steroid therapy in the immunosuppressed. Consider whether steroids are to be used on a case by case basis, depending on age, severity of pain, and degree of immunosuppression. If administered to these patients give them with acyclovir.

MANAGEMENT OF ACUTE HERPES ZOSTER PAIN

1. Topical therapy with drying soaks followed by application of silver sulfadiazine or lidocaine ointment may provide mild benefit. For thoracic and extremity lesions an Ace wrap to cover the involved area may significantly reduce the discomfort.
2. Acetaminophen, salicylates, and NSAIDs are sometimes adequate, and may be tried initially. The latter two agents may induce hemorrhage into the blisters. Add codeine if these are not satisfactory.
3. Systemic corticosteroids are sometimes beneficial and may be used in the nonimmunosuppressed patient.
4. Acyclovir may reduce the acute pain, especially if given intravenously. For the hospitalized patient, severe pain is an indication for intravenous acyclovir.
5. Amitriptyline beginning at 25 mg q.h.s. and increasing by 25 mg q.h.s. every other night to a maximum of 75 mg q.h.s. is often of great benefit. This may be the best oral therapy for acute and chronic zoster neuralgia.
6. Intradermal injections in the involved area with a long-acting anesthetic (bupivacaine 0.25%) may reduce acute pain. This therapy may be combined with sublesional triamcinolone (see below).
7. Dilute triamcinolone acetonide (2 mg/cc) injected sublesionally may provide acute relief. The treatment may need to be repeated q.d. for up to 2 weeks. Up to 30 cc of solution (60 mg of triamcinolone) may be used for each treatment. This is a significant dose of systemic steroid and physicians must be conscious of potential steroid side effects.
8. Even a brief respite from the pain is welcomed by the patient, and often when the pain returns it is much less severe. Early referral of patients with severe pain to an anesthesiologist or a pain clinic for a nerve block, ganglion block, or epidural block is extremely rewarding.

Alternative Therapy

1. Intravenous vidaribine 10 mg/kg/day may be used, but is not as effective as intravenous acyclovir.
2. Intramuscular triamcinolone acetonide 40 mg/week for 3 weeks may be used instead of oral corticosteroids for the prevention of postherpetic neuralgia.
3. Intramuscular ACTH 1mg/day for 2 weeks is an alternative to oral or intramuscular corticosteroids.

Subsequent Therapy

Patients given acyclovir are evaluated after 5–6 days of therapy. If no new lesions have occurred over the last 24–48 hours, those on intravenous therapy may be switched to oral therapy in full doses for a total of 10 days of therapy. For those with visceral dissemination a total of 7 days of intravenous therapy is indicated. For those begun on oral acyclovir continue the therapy for 7 days if there are no new lesions after 3 full days of treatment, and for 10 days if new lesions occurred after 3 days of therapy.

Pitfalls

1. Occasionally herpes simplex will appear in a zosteriform pattern. Culture these lesions or examine them by fluorescent antibody, especially if recurrent, as the acyclovir dosage requirements are different.
2. Begin acyclovir therapy as soon as possible (within the first 96 hours of the eruption).
3. Acyclovir has few side effects if administered correctly:
   a. Correct the dosage for the patient's renal function.
   b. Adequately hydrate the patient (1 L of fluid/dose of acyclovir).
   c. Infuse the acyclovir slowly (over 1–2 hours).
   d. Monitor the patient's renal function during therapy and correct the dose for changes in renal functin.
   e. Dilute the acyclovir sufficiently (6 mg/ml or less).
4. Due to its poor bioavailability, oral acyclovir has not been reported to alter renal function. It also does not reach the tissue levels that guarantee treatment of all strains of herpes zoster. For those with dissemination or those at high risk for dissemination, intravenous acyclovir must be used.

POSTHERPETIC NEURALGIA

Many of the therapies effective for acute zoster pain are also effective for postherpetic neuralgia.

Initial Therapy

1. Topical capsaicin (Zostrix) applied 5×day may reduce the pain after several weeks of treatment.
2. Amitryptyline beginning at 25 mg q.h.s. and increasing slowly up to 100 mg q.h.s. appears to be the most effective single oral agent.

Subsequent Therapy

1. Intralesional therapy with bupivacaine with or without triamcinolone acetonide (2 mg/cc) is often adjunctively useful in pain management.
2. Nerve blocks, although short lived, may be useful in reducing the level of pain.
3. A phenothiazine may be added to the amitryptyline in patients not completely responding to the latter.
4. Refer those who have failed on all of the above treatments to a clinic specializing in pain management for consideration of transcutaneous electrical nerve stimulation (TENS), acupuncture, or surgery.

Pitfalls

1. Patients discontinuing capsaicin topically may note a rebounding of the pain. Taper the drug slowly.
2. These patients often require significant analgesia. Use caution when prescribing narcotics to avoid dependency.
3. Tricyclic antidepressants have many side effects. These may be more significant in the elderly with associated diseases, especially heart disease. They should be used with caution and careful monitoring.
4. Patients with thoracic zoster may splint because of pain, leading to atelectasis. Patients should be advised to adequately inflate their lungs. A nerve block may be required to allow this.

TB

89

Hidradenitis Suppurativa and Perifolliculitis Capitis

Perifolliculitis Capitis Abscedens et Suffoidiens • Dissecting Cellulitis of the Scalp

Hidradenitis suppurativa and perifolliculitis capitis are chronic inflammatory processes that affect the groin, axilla, and inframammary areas (hidradenitis suppurativa) and the scalp (dissecting cellulitis). Progression is often relentless and defies medical management. Early surgery for local and widespread lesions is often the best alternative.

Initial Therapy

MEDICAL

1. Culture draining sinus tracts or abscesses for aerobic and anaerobic bacteria.
2. Give full-dose oral antibiotics effective against the isolated organisms for 1 month. Tetracycline, amoxicillin, penicillin, dicloxacillin, cephalosporins, and clindamycin have all been used with variable results.
3. Prescribe topical clindamycin solution to be applied to the affected areas b.i.d.

SURGICAL

1. Incise and drain fluctuant abscesses.
2. Inject triamcinolone acetonide 5–10 mg/cc into all nonfluctuant inflammatory areas. This may be repeated at intervals of 2–4 weeks.
3. Local areas may be totally excised, if small, with good results.

Ancillary Therapy

1. Encourage obese patients with disease in the intertriginous areas to lose weight.
2. Oral zinc sulfate 220 mg t.i.d. may be beneficial. In one case of perifolliculitis capitis, complete healing resulted.

Subsequent Therapy

INITIAL POSITIVE RESPONSE

1. Continue oral antibiotics and taper them slowly over 6–12 months. If the disease recurs, reculture and repeat initial management.
2. Because relapse and persistence is the rule, even patients who have responded well to conservative therapy may be offered more extensive surgical procedures, especially for axillary disease (see below).

INITIAL TREATMENT FAILURE

1. Medical Treatment
   a. Systemic corticosteroids (prednisone 0.5–1 mg/kg/day) for several weeks will significantly reduce inflammation. When combined with appropriate antibiotics, corticosteroids may also allow the disease to be controlled.
   b. Isotretinoin 1–2 mg/kg has been effective in some patients. Large series have not been reported, but limited experience has shown that results are often disappointing, with the response rate being as low as 50% or less. Where there is no contraindication, a course should be attempted.
   c. For severe recalcitrant dissecting disease of the scalp, low-dose x-ray epilation (Adamson-Keibock technique) will usually at least temporaily control severe recalcitrant disease.
2. Surgical treatment
   Extensive surgical procedures usually offer the only hope for the severely affected.
   a. For axillary disease, total excision of the affected axillary areas is of only moderate morbidity and gives excellent results. After their convalescence, patients are in general quite happy with the long-term, usually permanent remission.
   b. Genitocrural hidradenitis can also be totally excised, but often extensive grafting or prolonged healing is required owing to the large areas of involvement. Despite this, after convalescence most patients are satisfied.

c. Total excision of the affected scalp in dissecting cellulitis of the scalp is also effective, and often curative. Patients are usually rendered permanently bald, so a hairpiece may be required.

Pitfalls

1. These disease processes are aggressive, and require aggressive management to obtain disease control.
2. For the side effects of isotretinoin and intralesional and systemic corticosteroids, see Appendices 4, 5 and 6.
3. Tetracycline is contraindicated in pregnancy.
4. With high-dose zinc sulfate, GI upset is common.
5. Patients face a two-fold risk of carcinoma in these conditions. If the disease is chronic, squamous cell carcinomas, which may be fatal, may occur. In addition, there is an increased risk of cutaneous carcinoma in the radiation treated areas, especially in Caucasians. Any suspicious nonhealing lesion requires biopsy.

TB

90

Hirsutism

The etiology of hirsutism may be familial, idiopathic, drug-induced, or part of an androgen-excess sydrome.

Initial Therapy and Work-Up

1. A thorough history and physical examination are required to exclude virilization syndromes. Even in the absence of positive findings, obtain minimal laboratory screening tests, including serum/plasma DHEAS, free testosterone, androstenedione, prolactin, free cortisol, 11-deoxycortisol (compound S), and 17-hydroxyprogesterone. This battery will exclude ovarian, adrenal, and pituitary causes of hyperandrogenemia. If any abnormalities are encountered, the patient should consult an endocrinologist for further work-up.
2. The list of systemic drugs that induce hair growth is growing. The clinician

needs to assess for such potential offenders as steroid hormones, phenothiazines, minoxidil, triamterene-hydrochlorothiazide (Dyazide), dilantin, acetazolamide (Diamox), penicillamine, and psoralens.

3. For minor adrenal androgen overactivity:
   a. A low-dose corticosteroid regimen can be employed (e.g., prednisolone 2.5 mg q.a.m. and 5.0 mg q.h.s); or
   b. Spironolactone (Aldactone) 100 mg/day, increasing gradually to 100 mg q.i.d. if no change occurs in 12–16 weeks. Both steroids and spironolactone will slowly reduce hirsutism, but long-term maintenance is required for at least 2 years.

4. For ovarian androgen hyperactivity: Prescribe cyclic estrogen-dominant OCPs (e.g., ethinylestradiol plus ethinodiol (Demulen)). *Note:* Estrogens also are useful for androgen-dominant hirsutism.

5. Cosmetic therapy:
   a. Shaving is useful and does not (contrary to popular belief) stimulate hair growth, nor does it change the character of hairs. However, it may be psychologically unacceptable for many women.
   b. Epilation, by manual plucking or waxing, is useful for limited areas of excess hair growth, but may be irritating. Moreover, epilation usually needs to be repeated every 6 weeks.
   c. Bleaching is useful ancillary therapy because it decreases the frequency with which hair-removal methods need be employed.

Alternative Therapy

1. Ketoconozole possesses mild antiandrogen activity. Doses of 200 mg b.i.d. have been employed for the treatment of hirsutism, with at least 6 months required for a response to be observed.
2. Cimetidine 300 mg b.i.d. has mild antiandrogen activity, and can reduce excessive hair growth.
3. Topical antiandrogens are not yet available in the United States, but are effective and several will reach the marketplace in the near future.
4. Electrolysis is the only effective method for permanent hair removal, but should not be used initially for reasons described in Pitfalls, below.
5. Depilatory creams containing calcium thioglycollate, despite their ready availability, should be avoided because of their irritant and sensitizing potential.

Pitfalls

1. It is imperative that a neoplastic cause of hirsutism be sought and excluded in the work-up of hirsutism.

2. Some estrogen-containing OCPs (e.g., norethindrone) also contain substantial progesterone, which actually can aggravate hirsutism. In addition, the possible vascular and embolic side effects of estrogen-dominant OCPs should be monitored carefully in patients on these agents.
3. Electrolysis is somewhat painful, expensive, can aggravate acne, and can leave focal scars if done improperly. Refer patients only to a reputable, licensed electrologist if this therapy is desired.
4. Epilation can reactivate orolabial herpes simplex.

PE

91

Histiocytosis X Syndromes

Langerhans' Cell Histiocytoses

Histiocytosis X syndromes are a group of disorders most common in childhood. Their course varies from localized (bone, skin, and rarely, other organs) and benign, to severe and fatal, with internal organ involvement. Involvement and dysfunction of lungs, liver, and/or bone marrow are very poor prognostic signs. Skin-limited cases and sometimes systemic disease may spontaneously involute without therapy. Disease may recur after involution, even years later, therefore long-term follow-up is essential. Histiocytosis X syndromes are uncommon, and most patients should be evaluated and usually managed at tertiary referral centers.

A staging system accurately determines which patients require and benefit from chemotherapy (see JM Lipton: The pathogenesis, diagnosis and treatment of histiocytosis syndromes. *Pediatric Dermatology* 1:112–120, 1983). Therapy is individualized to the patient's extent of disease and its effect on organ systems. Needless chemotherapy-induced morbidity should be avoided, with no or only local therapy for local disease. A biopsy of affected tissue for diagnoses should be performed. Evaluation for internal organ involvement includes bone radiographs, CBC with platelets, LFTs, liver-spleen scan, bone marrow biopsy (if the CBC is abnormal), and urinalysis and serum electrolytes (to look for diabetes insipidus).

CUTANEOUS-ONLY DISEASE

Initial Therapy

Patients may be observed without therapy. Autoinvolution usually occurs.

Alternative Therapy

1. Topical nitrogen mustard has cleared cutaneous lesions in adults and children. Dosage and application are similar to those used in cutaneous T-Cell Lymphoma (see Ch. 39). Concentrations from 2% to 10% in saline are applied q.d. until the eruption clears (usually in 2–4 weeks). Weekly or biweekly maintenance may be required.
2. PUVA and UVB therapy have been used in several patients with good results. Maintenance may be required.
3. Prednisone alone may be used for extensive cutaneous disease. For severe disease single-agent chemotherapy may be considered (see below).

SOLITARY BONE LESIONS

Initial Therapy

Curettage or intralesional steroid injections are highly effective, with complete resolution of lesions within 3 years.

Subsequent Therapy

Radiation therapy is also efficacious, but the long-term sequelae must be considered. Administration of 450–900 rads (up to 1,500 for large lesions) in 200-rad fractions may be utilized. Lesions recurring after injection or curettage may be radiated.

MULTIPLE BONE LESIONS WITH NO ORGAN INVOLVEMENT

Initial Therapy

Steroid injections to lesions.

Subsequent Therapy

If lesions continue to progress add chemotherapy (see below).

INTERNAL ORGAN INVOLVEMENT

Initial Therapy

Accurately stage the patient, and consult with a tertiary referral center or an experienced pediatric oncologist. Initially, use the most benign chemotherapeutic protocols (e.g., vinblastine-prednisone) with trials of more aggressive protocols (e.g., vincristine-prednisone-methotrexate or methotrexate-6-mercaptopurine) should the disease fail to respond. Although chlorambucil is an effective agent, second malignancies have occurred in 10% of patients treated at one center with this agent. Use it after other agents have failed.

Pitfalls

1. Congenital self-healing reticulohistiocytosis is a benign Langerhans' cell histiocytosis almost identical to histiocytosis X clinically and histologically. This diagnosis should be entertained in neonates with lesions over 1 cm and skin involvement only. As the name implies, autoinvolution occurs universally by 3 months.
2. Severe combined immunodeficiency syndrome and graft vs. host disease may closely mimic histiocytosis X. In histiocytosis X most patients are reasonably immunologically normal prior to therapy when evaluated by standard tests.
3. Morbidity and mortality may be reduced by appropriate nonaggressive therapy (often no therapy). Do not produce unnecessary permanent sequelae from overaggressive local or systemic treatments.
4. The side effects of PUVA and UVB therapy are discussed in Chapter 147, Psoriasis.

5. The side effects of topical nitrogen mustard are discussed in Chapter 39, Cutaneous T-Cell Lymphoma.
6. Long-term follow-up is essential to detect disease relapse and to monitor for long-term complications (cosmetic, orthopaedic, hearing impairment, loss of permanent teeth, pulmonary fibrosis, cor pulmonale, portal hypertension, cirrhosis, endocrinologic disorders from pituitary involvement, and second malignancies from radiation therapy and chemotherapy).

TB

92

Hymenoptera Stings

Bee • Wasp • Hornet Stings

Hymenoptera stings cause toxic and allergic reactions. Toxic reactions can be mild when the stings are few, or severe and fatal if many stings occur. Allergic responses can be local exaggerated reactions or a generalized systemic reaction.

TOXIC REACTIONS

Initial Therapy

1. Remove all embedded stingers as promptly as possible, as venom continues to be injected after the stinger is detached from the insect. Do not squeeze or pick up the stinger with fingers; instead, scrape laterally with a blade or use a fine tweezers.
2. Apply ice (not heat) early, and elevate and rest the affected extremity.
3. For severe reactions, analgesia and sedation may be required.
4. Intravenous calcium gluconate 10% solution 10 ml may benefit patients with severe toxic reactions. Infusions may need to be repeated at 1–4-hour intervals.

Subsequent Therapy

For severe toxic reactions, carefully observe the patient until stable. Hospitalization may be required. Toxic reaction can be fatal. For a nonsensitized adult, about 500 stings may inject a lethal dose of venom.

Pitfalls

Administer intravenous calcium gluconate only while vital signs and cardiac rhythm are monitored.

ALLERGIC REACTIONS

In *local exaggerated reactions* onset of persistent and exaggerated swelling of the sting site or contiguous areas may be immediate or delayed (24–48 hours). Although positive skin tests and elevated venom-specific IgE antibodies are found in patients with local exaggerated reactions, they tend to wane, and repeat stings infrequently result in systemic reactions.

Generalized allergic reactions are IgE-mediated systemic reactions and are similar to systemic allergic drug reactions. They range from a few urticarial lesions to anaphylactic shock. Death may result from respiratory compromise or vascular collapse.

Initial Therapy

LOCAL EXAGGERATED REACTION

1. Manage as stated above for toxic reactions; remove stingers, elevate, apply ice, and rest affected area.
2. Antihistamines in full doses (diphenhydramine or hydroxyzine 50 mg q.6h.) may be helpful, especially if given as soon as the reaction begins.
3. For persistent severe local reactions, a short course of systemic corticosteroids (prednisone) beginning at 1 mg/kg or 60 mg/day will hasten the resolution of the reaction.

GENERALIZED ALLERGIC REACTION

1. For mild reactions, oral histamines and an inhaled bronchodilator (e.g., epinephrine HCl aerosol) may be adequate.

2. For moderate to severe reactions, manage as anaphylaxis. (Refer to a standard textbook of emergency or internal medicine.)
3. Remove any embedded stingers.

Subsequent Therapy

LOCAL EXAGGERATED REACTION

1. Refer the patient to an allergist. Sensitization immunotherapy may be considered.
2. A Medic-Alert bracelet may be indicated.

GENERALIZED ALLERGIC REACTION

1. Referral to an allergist is recommended.
2. The patient should wear a Medic-Alert bracelet and carry an emergency kit containing antihistamines, a bronchodilator, and an epinephrine injection.
3. Educate the patient on how to avoid being stung (i.e., know and avoid areas where hymenoptera live and feed; avoid attractants (cosmetics, perfumes, bright-colored "flowery" clothing, and long loose hair); and remove nests from the local environment (severely allergic individuals should not do this themselves)).

Pitfalls

1. Local reactions around the mouth or throat may lead to respiratory compromise without a systemic allergic component. Carefully observe these patients.
2. Local exaggerated reactions around the eyes may be complicated by severe ophthalmic sequelae (e.g., atrophy of the iris, cataract, globe perforation, or glaucoma). If eye symptoms develop acutely or later, refer the patient to an ophthalmologist.
3. Local bacterial infection (cellulitis) may closely simulate the clinical picture of a local exaggerated reaction (see Ch. 24, Cellulitis).

TB

93

Hyperhidrosis

Idiopathic, essential or primary hyperhidrosis (with no underlying cause) of the palms, soles, and in the axillae is discussed.

Initial Therapy

1. Aluminum chloride 20% in anhydrous ethanol (Drysol) is the preferred initial therapy. It must be used carefully and exactly. Written patient instructions are suggested as follows:
   a. The skin must be totally dry before application. Use a blow-dryer in the axillae if necessary. Do not apply for 24–48 hours after shaving. In the axillae, apply only to the hairy area.
   b. Apply q.h.s. to take advantage of reduced nocturnal sweating. It must remain on for 6–8 hours.
   c. Wash off aluminum chloride in the morning.
   d. If axillary irritation results, apply hydrocortisone 1% cream b.i.d.
   e. If irritation persists despite use of hydrocortisone cream, reduce the concentration to 6.25% (Xerac AC).
   f. If nightly treatment for 1–2 weeks has not reduced sweating, occlude the aluminum chloride with gloves (palms) or plasticwrap (axillae, soles). For the axillae, put a rolled-up sock on top of the plastic wrap in the axillary vault, and wear a slightly small T-shirt. This may increase efficacy and decrease irritation.
2. For plantar hyperhidrosis, recommend to the patient nonocclusive footwear (leather shoes, cotton socks) and absorbent foot powder. Alternating pairs of shoes to allow previously worn shoes to thoroughly dry is also useful.

Alternative Therapy

1. Glutaraldehyde 2%–10% may be used on the soles. It will stain the skin brown.
2. Methenamine (a formaldehyde releaser) has also been reported to be effective topically. Avoid formaldehyde as it is a common sensitizer.

Subsequent Therapy

1. Initial improvement: Maintain aluminum chloride or glutaraldehyde treatment at once or twice weekly.
2. Initial failures:
   a. Iontophoresis: Use of a galvanic generator delivering 15–30 mA or a commercially available Drionic device delivering 20 mA is effective. Tap water treatment beginning at 20 minutes three to six times weekly gives good control. Treatment courses are repeated as needed.
   b. Glycopyrrolate and other anticholinergics benefit, but often the dose required causes too many side effects to be tolerated for long term.
   c. Surgery
      1. Axillae: The area of maximum sweating usually correlates with the hair-bearing area, but prior to surgery the hyperhidrotic area should be mapped. Excision into the fat of this area with primary closure usually gives good results without significant complications. A spread scar results. Heavy sweating may require a second procedure, removing additional axillary skin.
      2. Palms and soles: Surgery (i.e., upper thoracic sympathectomy) for palmar hyperhidrosis is a major undertaking, and is therefore reserved for the most refractory cases after extensive counselling. Although virtually all patients initially obtain relief, the sweating returns to some degree after a period. Compensatory hyperhidrosis of the nondenervated areas may occur. Lumbar sympathectomy may be associated with impotence, and should be avoided in treating plantar hyperhidrosis.
   d. Biofeedback training and psychotherapy have been reported to be effective.

TB

94

Ichthyosis

Ichthyosis results from abnormal retention and/or production of the stratum corneum layer of the epidermis. Acquired ichthyosis can be a cutaneous manifestation of an underlying disease (e.g., malignant neoplasm, metabolic disorder, malabsorption). The genetic ichthyoses comprise a heterogeneous group of disorders that are either limited to the skin (primary ichthyoses) or part of a systemic or developmental disease complex (e.g., Sjögren–Larsson syndrome, Refsum's disease). Not only are these disorders diverse in etiology, but the extent of scaling is variable as well, ranging from mild to severe. Thus, management is separated here into the therapy of mild and severe disease.

MILD ICHTHYOSIS

Initial Therapy

Emollients with added debriding agents, hydroxy acids, or hygroscopic agents are usually tried first: ammonium lactate 12% gel (Lac-Hydrin), lactic acid 6% lotion (LactiCare), aquaphor (Eucerin) cream with 5%–10% lactic acid if more emolliency is needed. They are applied q.d. immediately after bathing, while skin is still damp.

Alternative Therapy

Hydrated petrolatum with 6% lactic acid, 40% propylene glycol in water applied overnight under a space suit or Sleep Sauna, or hydrated petrolatum ointment with 10%–20% urea are useful alternatives in some patients.

Ancillary Therapy

Most milder forms of ichthyosis are accompanied by a relative inability of the skin to retain moisture. Therefore, the following measures should be employed in conjunction with all other types of therapy.

1. Oilated baths (e.g., Domol, Keri, or oilated colloidal oatmeal (Aveeno)) 1/2 cup/bath q.d.
2. Cool-water bathing in general will result in less delipidization, and hence, better water retention of the stratum corneum.
3. Mild soaps: Dove is the least expensive of currently available, mild soaps. Many other more expensive glycerinated or nonglycerinated, oilated soaps are equally effective.

Subsequent Therapy

1. The inherited ichthyoses are life-long diseases, and therapy should be adjusted for maximum patient convenience.
2. The hydroxy acids (i.e., lactic acid lotion, ammonium lactate gel, or glycolic acid lotion (Aquaglycolic acid)) are especially efficacious in recessive X-linked ichthyosis, and may be the only specific therapy needed for this disease.
3. Patients with acquired ichthyosis need to be evaluated for associated systemic diseases.
4. Exacerbations in winter and remissions in summer are the rule for the milder forms of ichthyosis, and therapy should be adjusted accordingly.

SEVERE FORMS OF ICHTHYOSIS

Severe forms of ichthyosis generally require the same topical approaches as milder forms. However, in addition, systemic retinoids may be indicated. Because the doses required for successful control of bullous ichthyosis (epidermolytic hyperkeratosis), lamellar ichthyosis, and congenital ichthyosiform erythroderma generally are higher than those employed for other applications (e.g., acne, cancer chemoprevention, or psoriasis), acute side effects can be more severe. Moreover, the benefits of improvement of the skin must be weighed against long-term risks (see Appendix 7). Finally, in prepubertal children there is the additional risk of premature closure of the epiphyses.

Initial Therapy

Etretinate or acitretin 1–2 mg/kg/day or isotretinoin 2–4 mg/kg/day; initial therapy should be at the lower dose levels indicated. *Note:* Systemic retinoids should be administered by physicians thoroughly acquainted with the indications and side effects of these agents.

Subsequent Therapy

1. Improvement should be evident within 6 weeks. If no change has occurred, the dose can be increased. If and when dramatic improvement has occurred, attempts should be made to reduce the dosage, and/or to employ q.o.d. therapy.

2. Topical therapy should be pursued aggressively throughout to allow reduction in total dosage of systemic retinoids.
3. Patients on long-term systemic retinoid therapy require monitoring of several blood parameters, as well as sequential radiographic studies (see Appendix 6). Retinoid therapy is best managed by a physician with special expertise in the applications and side effects of these drugs.

PE

95

Impetigo

The two major forms of impetigo, bullous impetigo and impetigo contagiosum, can masquerade as noninfectious diseases, both because of their lack of characteristic signs of acute infection (i.e., dolor, calor, rubor, tumor), and because of their tendency to form dry crusts. Moreover, both forms can complicate pre-existing dermatoses (e.g., eczemas, insect bites). The clustering of lesions around facial orifices and/or exposed areas of the body is an important diagnostic clue. The presence of yellowish crusts vs. annular erosions with minimal crusting distinguishes impetigo contagiosum from bullous impetigo. Although earlier studies suggested that the primary pathogen in impetigo contagiosum is *S. pyogenes*, lesions commonly become colonized with *S. aureus*, and therapy is best directed at both. Bullous impetigo is invariably due to *S. aureus*, usually phage group II, type 55 or 71 (elaborators of epidermolytic toxin; see Ch. 104, Staphylococcal Scalded Skin Syndrome).

Initial Therapy

1. Dicloxacillin 250 mg q.i.d. for 10 days.
2. Erythromycin 250 mg q.i.d. for 10 days is the preferred initial choice in penicillin-allergic individuals, although 15%–20% of strains of staphylococci are resistant to erythromycin.

Alternative Therapy

1. A cephalosporin, such as cephalexin 250 mg q.i.d. for 10 days.
2. Recent studies suggest that pseudomonic acid cream (Bactroban), applied t.i.d. to infected lesions, is as effective as systemic therapy for impetigo contagiosum.

Ancillary Therapy

1. Obtain culture and sensitivity of exudate.
2. Debridement of crusts, although commonly recommended, is probably unnecessary.
3. Impetigo tends to occur in mini-epidemics, especially within families, where nasal carriage of pathogens is common. Hence, family members and/or other cohabitants should treat the nasal vestibule with bacitracin or Neosporin ointment, applied with a Q-Tip, q.d. for 10 days, and shower with either chlorhexidine (Hibiclens) or povidone-iodine (Betadine) q.d. for 10 days. Individuals or families with persistent nasal carriage should be treated with dicloxacillin 250 mg q.i.d. plus rifampicin 300 mg b.i.d. for 7 days.
4. As infection responds, any underlying dermatitis, if present, should also be treated (see appropriate chapter).

Pitfalls

1. Reinfections, transmission within families, and persistent nasal carriage are common.
2. Transmission of phage group II or other epidermolytic toxin-generating strains of staphylococci to susceptible individuals (neonates, immunosuppressed individuals, persons in renal failure) rarely can result in more generalized forms of staphylococcal scalded skin syndrome.
3. Epidemics of nephritogenic strains of staphylococci can occur. Aggressive therapy is indicated to eliminate such organisms from the community.

PE

96

Ingrown Nail

Ingrown nails almost always involve the large toe (hallux). They are due to improper trimming of the nail and/or improperly fitting footwear, with overgrowth of granulation tissue and secondary bacterial infection.

Initial Therapy

1. If severe, partial or complete nail avulsion may be required.
2. If mild, taping the lateral nailfold tissue to pull it away from the nail may allow the trapped nail fragment to grow out.
3. Prescribe oral dicloxacillin 250 mg q.i.d. for 10 days.
4. Instruct patient on proper trimming of nails: do not trim too short; trim nails straight across.

Alternative Therapy

For chronic ingrown nails, avulsion plus ablation of the nail matrix may be the best long-term solution.

Pitfalls

A cutaneous malignancy may mimic a chronically ingrown toenail.

TB

97

Intestinal Bypass Dermatitis–Arthritis Syndrome

Bowel Bypass Syndrome

Intestinal bypass dermatitis is an episodic, circulating immune complex disease that occurs in about 20% of patients who have had ileojejunal bypass surgery. Cryoproteins are present, possibly directed against bacterial peptidoglycans. Other forms of bowel disease may be associated with a similar dermatosis-arthritis syndrome.

Initial Therapy

1. A broad-spectrum antibiotic, such as tetracycline 500 mg q.i.d., oral minocycline 100 mg q.d. to b.i.d., or metronidazole up to 1.5 g/day, will often abort attacks if begun early, and will often prevent attacks if taken chronically.
2. Adjunctively acetysalicylic acid (aspirin), phenylbutazone, or other NSAIDs may improve or control the arthritic symptoms.

Alternative Therapy

Oral sulfapyridine 500 mg q.i.d. or oral dapsone 100 mg q.d. to bid may be used as in other cutaneous vasculitides (see Ch. 104, Leukocytoclastic Vasculitis).

Subsequent Therapy

1. Patients who fail to respond to the above therapies often respond to chronic low-dose oral prednisone (10–20 mg/day).
2. When all the above medical therapies fail, surgical procedures, such as a sphincteroplasty, may control symptoms. Restoration of normal bowel anatomy is curative.

TB

98

Kaposi's Sarcoma

Kaposi's sarcoma (KS) occurs in four settings: classic KS, African KS, immunosuppressive-associated KS, and HIV-infection-associated (AIDS-associated) KS. The therapy of each form is discussed separately.

CLASSIC KAPOSI'S SARCOMA

Classic KS affects primarily elderly males of Mediterranean or Eastern European Jewish extraction. Although visceral involvement is found in up to 70% of patients (primarily in the GI tract), this is usually asymptomatic, and only 20% of patients with classic KS die of their disease. For this reason, therapy is often palliative and directed at control of local symptoms. Progressive disease may require more aggressive therapy.

Initial Therapy

1. For localized or limited disease, local or extended-field radiotherapy is highly efficacious. Doses as low as 800 rads may be effective in a single dose. Fractionated doses at 1,200–3,000 rads are also effective. Extended field radiotherapy will control edema as well as local lesions.
2. Solitary or a few lesions may be treated with local destruction by cryotherapy or intralesional injections with vinblastine or vincristine 0.2–0.5 mg/ml.
3. Lymphedema may precede or accompany KS. Control of the lymphedema with elevation and support stockings is important for patients with lower-extremity lesions. Ulceration and secondary infection are not infrequent, and require aggressive therapy with antibiotics and local dressings.
4. For debilitating extensive cutaneous disease, symptomatic visceral involvement, and relapses after radiation therapy, systemic chemotherapy with single agents (vinblastine or vincristine) or combinations (Adriamycin, bleomycin, vincristine) may be useful.

AFRICAN KAPOSI'S SARCOMA

African KS occurs in three forms in adults and children: localized cutaneous disease, localized aggressive disease (which may extend to underlying bone), and generalized disease. In areas endemic for HIV infection, AIDS-associated KS also occurs (see below).

Initial Therapy

1. Localized cutaneous disease is managed like localized classic KS, with radiotherapy or local vinca alkaloids injection.
2. Localized aggressive disease and generalized disease require systemic chemotherapy. The most commonly used agents are vincristine or vinblastine alone, or in combination with actinomycin D or imidazole carboxamide (DTIC). Unfortunately, most African KS patients present with quite advanced disease. Amputation is often required in patients with local cutaneous or locally aggressive disease.

IMMUNOSUPPRESSIVE-ASSOCIATED KAPOSI'S SARCOMA

Iatrogenic immunosuppression for connective tissue disease, malignancy (myeloma), or organ transplantation has been associated with the development of KS.

Initial Therapy

1. For localized disease, local measures such as radiation therapy, cryotherapy, or intralesional vinca alkaloid injections (see above) are effective.
2. Reduce the doses of immunosuppressive agents to the minimum required. If immunosuppressives can be significantly reduced or discontinued, the KS may regress.

Subsequent Therapy

Progressive, disseminated life-threatening KS may be treated with systemic chemotherapy (see above). This is difficult in the already-immunosuppressed individual.

AIDS-ASSOCIATED KS

Kaposi's sarcoma may occur as an initial or later complication of HIV infection. It may appear in patients with a relatively high helper T-cell count and no other evidence of immunosuppression, or in those with advanced HIV disease. In the terminal phase of HIV infection, KS may progress rapidly. Improvement of the overall health of the patient associated with AZT treatment or therapy of underlying infectious disease may lead to improvement or resolution of KS lesions. Visceral involvement is common, but often asymptomatic, and does not require therapy. Pulmonary KS appears to be more likely life-threatening and serious consideration should be given to treating it. Above all, the overall health of the patient must be considered in treating KS associated with AIDS. Therapy is palliative, not curative, so a priority system must be devised in managing the patient. Since KS is rarely life-threatening, other problems may need to be managed first. Therapy of the KS is not required except when potentially life-threatening.

Initial Therapy

1. Establish the diagnosis. Skin lesions are an excellent source of diagnostic material. Biopsy the thickest nonulcerated lesion. Punch, excision, or shave biopsies (of exophytic nodules) are adequate. Do *not* biopsy at the edge of skin lesions, but rather in the center.
2. Evaluate the overall status of the patient. Determine the level of immunosuppression, and look for HIV-associated infections and complications. Treat any treatable conditions.
3. Determine the extent and rate of progression of the HIV-associated KS. The following staging system may be used:
   Stage I: Localized cutaneous (fewer than 10 lesions, or one anatomic region);
   Stage II: Disseminated cutaneous (more than 10 lesions, or more than one anatomic area);
   Stage III: Visceral only;
   Stage IV: Cutaneous and visceral or pulmonary.
   The above stages may be further classified using these subtypes:
   Subtype A: No signs or symptoms;
   Subtype B: Systemic symptoms (fever or weight loss).
4. Because therapy is expensive, look for investigational studies for which the patient might qualify.

5. For stable cutaneous disease stages I and II, A or B
    a. Intralesional vinblastine or vincristine 0.2–0.5 mg/cc. Use 0.1–0.5 cc/lesion, not to exceed 2 mg/treatment session. Treatments may be repeated biweekly.
    b. For flat (macular) or slightly infiltrated lesions, especially those less than 1 cm in maximum diameter, cryotherapy with two freeze-thaw cycles (20–30 seconds thaw time) may be efficacious. Cryotherapy will also treat the residuae of lesions following radiation therapy or intralesional injection. Several treatments may be required for each lesion.
    c. Alternatively, radiation therapy is quite effective in a single dose of 800 rads or fractionated in doses of 1,000–3,000 rads. This is especially useful for painful or disfiguring lesions of the feet, penis, or face.
    d. Subsequently, for patients with stage II-A disease and helper T-cell counts over $200/mm^3$, intramuscular or subcutaneous α_2 interferon 30×10^6 IU/m^2 3×/week results in tumor regression in slightly over 50% of patients.
6. For localized lymphatic and mucosal disease, radiation therapy in fractionated doses may help control lymph node disease and the associated lymphedema. Patients with mucosal disease may require significant fractionation, as mucositis is a common complication of oropharyngeal radiation therapy for AIDS-associated KS.
7. For systemic, visceral, or pulmonary disease stages II-B, III-A,B, and IV-A,B, single-agent chemotherapy with vinca alkaloids or combination chemotherapy (Adriamycin, bleomycin, vincristine) is effective. Patients without systemic symptoms (subgroup A) have a much higher response rate. Immunosuppressive effects of these agents are a significant concern. Toxicity often limits therapy.

Pitfalls

1. Confirm KS by tissue biopsy, especially if skin lesions are present. KS is *not* a clinical diagnosis.
2. KS is rarely life-threatening, and therapy is palliative. Do not interfere with the overall health of the patient by overzealous treatment of KS.
3. Cryotherapy may lead to local scarring and hypopigmentation.
4. Large lesions of KS injected with vinca alkaloids may ulcerate. Ulcerated lesions heal with scarring.
5. Hyperpigmentation may occur after vinca alkaloid injections. Cryotherapy will reduce this side effect.

6. α-Interferon therapy frequently produces systemic symptoms (fever, chills, myalgias); these are transient.
7. The side effects of chemotherapeutic agents are discussed in Appendix 7.

TB

99

Keloids and Hypertrophic Scars

Keloids follow injury to the skin from a variety of causes. Sites of predilection are the ears, upper back and chest, and upper arms. Whereas hypertrophic scars involute by 6 months after their formation, keloids persist and even extend beyond the original margins. Keloids not only are disfiguring, but they also can exhibit the full spectrum from mild itch or tenderness to extreme hyperaesthesia.

Initial Therapy

Keloids can be softened progressively, and made less hyperaesthetic by injections of triamcinolone acetonide (Kenalog) 20 mg/cc directly into several adjacent sites within the lesion(s). Use a 25–30-gauge Luerlock needle and tuberculin syringe to allow injection under pressure. Give injections at monthly intervals until the desired degree of involution and/or symptomatic relief is achieved. If no change occurs after one injection with a concentration of 20 mg/cc, increase the dose to 40 mg/cc. If no change has occurred after three or four injections, consider surgical excision (see Alternative Therapy).

Alternative Therapy

If keloids do not respond or remain symptomatic, surgical excision is an alternative, although the lesions tend to recur (see Pitfalls). To avoid recurrences after excision, inject the base of the surgical site with triaminolone acetonide 20 mg/cc using a 30-gauge needle, in multiple sites along the excision site immediately after surgery, and occlude the excision site with a pressure dressing (e.g., Elastoplast). Injections then should be repeated at 2-week intervals over about 3–4 months. In addition, administer a short course of systemic steroids (over 10–14 days) if no contraindication to such therapy exists (see Appendix 5). Begin with 60 mg q.a.m. in a single oral dose with a meal or glass of milk, and taper over 10–14 days. *Note:* Because corticosteroids inhibit wound healing, the surgical site needs to be protected with a pressure dressing for the full course of therapy to avoid wound breakdown.

Pitfalls

1. Keloids tend to recur after excision, and can be very recalcitrant to all types of therapy. *Note:* Ears should not be repierced after excision of a prior keloid.
2. Recurrences can be more disfiguring than the original lesion, especially if relatively destructive, ablative methods such as electrosurgery are employed.
3. Because of the tendency of keloids to form in certain races, particularly blacks, elective surgery should be avoided.

PE

100

Keratoacanthoma

Keratoacanthomas (KA) are usually solitary, crateriform, rapidly growing squamoproliferative tumors occurring on the sun-exposed skin of elderly light-skinned patients. The natural history is one of spontaneous involution in less than 6 months in most cases. Multiple lesions can occur, occasionally in the familial setting.

Initial Therapy

For isolated lesions, surgical excision with minimal margins is usually curative and gives excellent cosmetic results.

Alternative Therapy

1. Intralesional injections of 5-fluorouracil (5-FU) 50 mg/cc to the crater edges and the base of the lesion often yields dramatic results. Inject a total of 0.5—1 cc of 5-FU once or twice weekly. After 2–3 weeks lesions are usually reduced by 70%. If not, a biopsy is required.
2. Patients with large or surgically difficult lesions and frail patients are good candidates for low-dose radiation therapy.
3. Patients with large numbers of KAs may be treated with oral retinoids (13-*cis* retinoic acid or etretinate). Chronic suppressive maintenance treatment may be required.

Subsequent Therapy

1. 5-FU therapy usually requires a total of 4–6 weeks of treatment.
2. Lesions failing to involute by 90% with intralesional 5-FU must be removed surgically or biopsied to rule out squamous cell carcinoma.

Pitfalls

1. In all but the most characteristic lesions, a biopsy is indicated to exclude squamous cell carcinoma.
2. KAs of the central face (nose and lips particularly) may be aggressive or persistent, and rarely show atypical histologic features (perineural and intravascular invasion). These lesions are best managed by those with experience in the treatment of KAs and cutaneous carcinomas.
3. For side effects of oral retinoids see Appendix 6. This therapy is contraindicated in females with child-bearing potential.

TB

101

Keratosis Pilaris

Keratosis pilaris (KP) is an extremely common, often dominantly inherited disorder that usually does not require treatment. Involvement of the face and upper arms, however, may be a significant cosmetic problem, and folliculitis not infrequently complicates KP on the buttocks and thighs.

Initial Therapy

1. If inflammatory lesions are present, an empiric trial of erythromycin or dicloxacillin 250 mg q.i.d. for 10 days is indicated.
2. A mild soap (e.g., Dove) or a soapless cleanser (e.g., Cetaphil) should be used with a mild abrasive scrub pad (e.g., Buf-Puf). This treatment will gradually remove follicular plugs (over several weeks) and prevent new ones from emerging.
3. Keralyt Gel (salicylic acid 6% in propylene glycol 40%) should be applied q.h.s. or after bathing. This therapy is particularly effective when used in conjunction with a Buf-Puf (see above).

Alternative Therapy

1. LacHydrin (ammonium lactate 12%) lotion is also effective for KP, and can be used in cases not responsive to Keralyt, or in addition to the latter.
2. Retinoic acid 0.025% cream q.h.s., increasing to 0.05% and 0.1%, as tolerated, may be helpful, but may be prohibitively expensive for the treatment of extensive disease.
3. A 3-month course of vitamin A palmitate (Aquasol A) 50,000 t.i.d. has been recommended by some authorities.

Subsequent Therapy

1. After the keratinous plugs have been removed, an emollient cream containing 20% urea (Carmol) may prevent reappearance of lesions.
2. Use of the abrasive scrub pad should be resumed at the first sign of reappearance of crops of new lesions.

3. A "dry skin program" of cool-to-tepid bathing, mild soaps, and lubrication also should be employed, as KP is almost invariably associated with xerosis (see Ch. 187), and may, in fact, predispose to exacerbations of KP.

Pitfalls

1. Both salicylic and lactic acids may be irritating, especially when applied to inflamed skin. A medium-potency, topical corticosteroid cream can be applied with these agents to reduce inflammation.
2. The side effects of topical retinoic acid are described in Chapter 2, Acne Vulgaris.
3. The side effects of oral vitamin A are comparable to, or even worse than, those of oral synthetic retinoids. Hence, therapy should be limited to 3-month bursts, and only employed after a pretreatment check of LFTs, cholesterol, and triglycerides. These laboratory parameters should then be rechecked monthly.

PE

102

Kyrle's Disease

Hyperkeratosis in Cutem Penetrans

Kyrle's disease, or hyperkeratosis in cutem penetrans, can be familial or acquired, as in chronic renal disease. Choice of therapy is dependent on the extent of involvement and/or degree of symptomatology.

Initial Therapy

LIMITED DISEASE

1. Applications of retinoic acid (Retin-A) 0.05% cream b.i.d. for 1–3 months, or until lesions resolve, is successful in about 50% of cases.
2. Liquid nitrogen cryosurgery is usually successful for the treatment of individual, recalcitrant lesions.

WIDESPREAD DISEASE

1. Although published information is still scanty, either etretinate (Tegison) 50–75 mg q.d., or acitretin 25–50 mg q.d., or isotretinoin (Accutane) 80–120 mg/day should eliminate lesions of Kyrle's disease. Because relapses are likely to occur after therapy is withdrawn, decrease the dosage slowly and stop therapy after 3–4 months, maintaining aggressive topical therapy for residual or recurrent lesions.

Alternative Therapy

1. A salicylic acid 6% gel (Keralyt) may be useful alone or in conjunction with topical retinoic acid.
2. Both local excision and/or electrodesiccation can be used for recalcitrant lesions.
3. Although both systemic methotrexate and topical 5-fluorouracil have been employed, their efficacy has not been demonstrated convincingly.

Pitfalls

1. Kyrle's disease can be a skin marker for underlying chronic renal disease; therefore, a work-up is appropriate.
2. The tendency for Kyrle's disease to relapse, even after successful therapy, has been noted above.
3. The side effects of systemic retinoids are detailed in Appendix 6.

PE

103

Leishmaniasis

As with all infectious diseases, the diagnosis of leishmaniasis should be established by identifying the causative agent in the affected tissue by culture, scrapings, or biopsy. Response to therapy is significantly related to the causative species and geographic area in which the infection was acquired. Leishmaniasis occurs in three forms: cutaneous, mucocutaneous, and visceral. Only the therapy of cutaneous leishmaniasis is discussed here.

OLD WORLD LEISHMANIASIS

The following therapy may not apply to disease acquired in Africa. Because mucocutaneous relapse is quite rare local therapy to the lesions alone is acceptable. The natural history is one of spontaneous healing without therapy. Treatment of lesions in cosmetically insignificant areas is not required.

Initial Therapy

Treatment is with paromomycin sulfate 15% and methylbenzethonium chloride 12% in white soft paraffin applied b.i.d. for 10 days.

Alternative Therapy

1. Chlorpromazine 2% ointment applied as above may also be effective.
2. Medical: Oral ketaconazole 400–1200 mg/day or rifampin (with or without isoniazid) 600–1200 mg/day until healed.
3. Surgical: Cryotherapy of individual lesions (forming an iceball 2 mm beyond the lesion). Local heat therapy 20 hours/day. Surgical excision of solitary small lesions may be curative.

Subsequent Therapy

Use antimonial therapy as discussed below for New World leishmaniasis in Old World cutaneous disease only when standard therapies fail and/or disease is progressive or disfiguring. Antimony potassium tartrate 10% cream has cleared some lesions, as has intralesional antimony.

Pitfalls

1. Oral ketoconazole may cause hepatitis. Monitor LFTs.
2. Oral rifampin will cause all body secretions to be colored reddish brown. Hepatitis and thrombocytopenia may occur. Rifampin reduces the efficacy of oral contraceptives.
3. Delay for at least 1 year after apparent complete healing any corrective plastic surgical procedures. During this period local relapse may occur, destroying any benefit gained by the surgical procedures.

NEW WORLD LEISHMANIASIS (AMERICAN LEISHMANIASIS)

Response to therapy is clearly species and subspecies related. Mucocutaneous disease is a potential and disastrous complication of New World leishmaniasis. Treat cases acquired in areas where mucocutaneous disease may occur with systemic agents (preferably antimonials).

Initial Therapy

1. Treat patients with extensive cutaneous lesions or cutaneous lesions acquired in an *L. braziliensis*-endemic area with systemic antimonials (i.e., intramuscular or intravenous sodium stibogluconate (Pentostam) 20 mg/kg for 20 days). N-Methylglucamine antimonate (Glucantime) 50–60 mg/kg/day may also be used. (Only Pentostam is available in the United States, and it must be obtained from the Centers for Disease Control.)
2. Patients with few lesions not acquired in an *L. braziliensis*-endemic area may be treated with ketoconazole 400–1200 mg/day till healed.

Alternative Therapy

Intralesional and topical antimonials also may be tried.

Subsequent Therapy

1. If the lesions have partially, but not completely responded after a single course of systemic antimonial therapy, a second (third, etc.) course may be given after a 10-day rest period.
2. Treat patients failing to respond to antimonial therapy with intravenous amphotericin B 0.5–1 mg/kg/dose to a total of 1.5–2.0 g.
3. Patients must be followed periodically for relapse.

Pitfalls

1. Antimonials are potentially quite toxic; electrocardiographic changes, renal and liver toxicities, vomiting, and myalgias may occur.
2. Amphotericin B is nephrotoxic; monitoring renal function and serum electrolytes (especially potassium) is required.

TB

104

Leukocytoclastic Vasculitis

In approximately 50% of cases, cutaneous leukocytoclastic vasculitis (LCV) is caused by associated disease or underlying infection, or by a chemical or drug. This therapeutic discussion assumes the cause of the remaining 50% is idiopathic. Because cutaneous LCV may be associated with internal organ involvement, this must be looked for in every patient. Treatment may be required for systemic disease even when skin lesions are mild.

Initial Therapy

The therapeutic goal is suppression or control of cutaneous lesions and symptoms. Because response to a given therapy is unpredictable, the clinician must choose from an empiric list of agents and be certain that the therapy employed is not more dangerous than the disease.

1. Treat with antihistamines; a combination of hydroxyzine (Atarax) 25–50 mg t.i.d. or q.i.d. and cyproheptadine 4 mg q.i.d. is occasionally useful. If the patient responds to this regimen, it may be continued as long as necessary.
2. Cutaneous ulcers or bullae may be treated with debridement, tap water compresses, and application of a semiocclusive dressing such as Duoderm or Restore.

Alternative Therapy

These therapeutic alternatives may be tried in individual cases until a therapeutic response is achieved or the disorder abates spontaneously; if the disorder recurs, choose another alternative.

1. No treatment; wait 2–3 weeks for spontaneous resolution.
2. Treat with prednisone 60 mg in daily or divided doses for 4–7 days. If the patient responds, taper prednisone over a 14-day period.
3. Treat with colchicine 0.6 mg t.i.d. Expect a response in 7–10 days.
4. Treat with dapsone 50 mg b.i.d. and increase the dose up to 100 mg b.i.d.

5. The success of azathioprine, cyclophosphamide, and methotrexate is unpredictable; they should be reserved only for the most severe cases or those with systemic disease.

Pitfalls

1. Do not overlook a treatable, underlying cause. Each patient must be fully evaluated and any potential causative drugs must be eliminated.
2. Evaluate for systemic involvement, especially renal (e.g., urinalysis with microscopic evaluation of urine sediment) and GI (e.g., stool guaiac).

BW

105

Lichen Myxedematosus

Scleromyxedema

Lichen myxedematosus is largely unresponsive to treatment, and available therapies have significant short-term and long-term complications. Therapy should be restricted to those with severe disease. Spontaneous resolution may occur.

Initial Therapy

1. Facial lesions may be improved with radiation therapy or dermabrasion. Gradual recurrence is to be anticipated.
2. Isotretinoin 1–2 mg/kg/day may be beneficial in some patients, as may etretinate or acitretin (Psoritane) 0.5–1 mg/kg/day.
3. Scleromyxedema may be associated with myeloma or a paraproteinemia. Look for it.

Subsequent Therapy

1. Patients should be followed for development of systemic disease.

2. If severe skin or systemic disease is present, melphalan beginning at 2 mg/day may be considered. Cyclophosphamide may also be beneficial.

Pitfalls

1. Scleromyxedema may involve internal organs, causing symptoms similar to those seen in scleroderma (e.g., dysphagia and restrictive lung disease). Regular evaluation for pulmonary, esophageal, or muscular involvement is advised.
2. Retinoids (isotretinoin, acitretin, and etretinate) should be administered only by those familiar with their frequent side effects (see Appendix 6). Pregnancy is absolutely contraindicated.
3. Immunosuppressive agents can cause marrow suppression, leading to leukopenia and subsequent infection. Melphalan therapy may be associated with the subsequent development of lymphoreticular malignancies. These agents should only be used by those experienced with them (see Appendix 6).

TB

106

Lichen Nitidus

Characterized by myriads of tiny flat-topped papules, lichen nitidus is thought by many to be related to lichen planus. As with lichen planus, the mainstay of therapy is topical steroids. The disease may spontaneously involute at any time.

Initial Therapy

1. Prescribe a high-potency steroid cream or gel (e.g., fluocinonide) to be applied b.i.d. for 1 month. If no response has occurred, a superpotent steroid cream or ointment can be tried q.d. for 1 month. *Note:* A low-potency preparation should be used for intertriginous or facial lesions.
2. For pruritus, which occurs only in a minority of patients, hydroxyzine 10 mg t.i.d. increasing to 25 mg q.i.d., if necessary, is usually effective.
3. An alternate strategy for pruritus is the use of a menthol-camphor-phenol-

containing lotion (e.g., Sarna) and/or oilated colloidal oatmeal (Aveeno) baths.

Alternate Therapy

1. Topical retinoic acid may be useful for the treatment of localized clusters of lesions. Prescribe retinoic acid 0.025% cream q.h.s. initially, increasing the concentration to 0.05 and 0.1% as tolerated, if response does not occur at a lower concentration.
2. Because isotretinoin (Accutane), etretinate (Tegison), and acitretin (Psoritane) have helped patients with widespread, recalcitrant lichen planus, a trial of these agents rarely may be indicated in some cases (see Ch. 107, Lichen Planus, for therapeutic guidelines).

Pitfalls

1. The pitfalls of topical steroids are described in Appendix 3.
2. The pitfalls of systemic retinoid therapy are described in Appendix 6.

TB

107

Lichen Planus

Lichen planus may be self-limited or chronic, and presents as localized or generalized disease, usually with mild to severe pruritus. Occasional patients have ulcerative, painful lesions. The aim of therapy is to control symptoms, and therefore must be appropriate to the extent and severity of the disease.

LOCALIZED LICHEN PLANUS

Initial Therapy

1. Apply superpotent fluorinated topical steroid ointment or cream q.d. to b.i.d. until the lesions flatten and disappear.

2. Prescribe an antihistamine to control pruritus. During waking hours, terfenadine (Seldane) 60–120 mg q.d. to b.i.d. may be taken. Before bed, diphenhydramine (Benadryl) 50–100 mg or hydroxyzine (Atarax) 25–50 mg may be taken.

Subsequent Therapy

1. Reduce the superpotent fluorinated topical steroid to a medium-potency agent (e.g., triamcinolone acetonide (Kenalog) 0.1% ointment or cream q.d. to b.i.d.), and apply as necessary to control lesions.
2. Reduce antihistamines to levels necessary to control pruritus.

Alternative Therapy

1. Occlude superpotent steroids with plastic wrap q.d. Occlusive dressings may be applied for 4–6 hours prior to bed, or overnight, if tolerated. When lesions flatten (within 7–14 days), discontinue occlusion and continue topical steroids alone as above.
2. Inject lesions with triamcinalone acetonide 5–10 mg/ml, and repeat in 2–3 weeks. One to three treatments per lesion are usually adequate.

GENERALIZED LICHEN PLANUS

Initial Therapy

Treat with oral prednisone (or an equivalent steroid) at 40–60 mg/day. Maintain the dose until symptoms abate and lesions clear.

Subsequent Therapy

Taper prednisone at a rate of 10 mg/week until a dose of 20 mg q.d. is reached, then taper by 5 mg/week. Expect recurrence when the dose reaches 20–30 mg/day, and control with topical steroids if possible. All patients will clear, but only about 25% will remain disease free. Patients who have a recurrence *must* be weaned from steroids. Other alternatives (see below) should be employed.

Alternative Therapy

1. Photochemotherapy (PUVA) may be helpful. Treat 3×/week and expect a response in 3–6 weeks.

2. Etretinate (Tegison) 0.5–1.0 mg/kg/day.
3. Isotretinoin (Accutane) 20–60 mg daily.

FOLLICULAR AND/OR NAIL LICHEN PLANUS

Treat as if disease were generalized. The scarring hair and nail loss is permanent, and an aggressive approach is reasonable in the absence of medical contraindications.

HYPERTROPHIC LICHEN PLANUS

Initial Therapy

1. Intralesional steroids (triamcinalone acetonide 10 mg/ml). Repeat weekly or bi-weekly if necessary.
2. Application of superpotent topical steroids (e.g., clobetasol propionate (Temovate or Diprolene)) with or without occlusion with plastic wrap. Occlusion of lesions for 4–10 hours.

Alternative Therapy

Those therapies listed for generalized lichen planus may be attempted, with or without topical steroids.

ORAL LICHEN PLANUS

Most nonulcerative cases are asymptomatic and do not require therapy. Ulcerative disease is often symptomatic, and should be treated.

Initial Therapy

1. Apply fluorinated steroids in a gelatin dental paste (Kenalog in Orabase) as frequently as possible.
2. Inject lesions with triamcinalone acetonide 5–10 mg/cc using a 30-gauge needle. Lesions may be injected every 2–3 weeks, up to 3–4 times if necessary.
3. Apply topical anesthetic (viscous lidocaine) as needed.

Subsequent Therapy

If symptoms cannot be controlled, systemic steroids, given as for widespread lichen planus, are appropriate.

Pitfalls

1. Lichen planus may be drug induced. Commonly used culprits include thiazides, gold, quinidine, and chloroquine. Discontinue these agents. In the case of gold-induced lichen planus, resolution may take months.
2. Most cases of lichen planus resolve spontaneously. Do not use long-term, chronic systemic steroid therapy to control lesions. Rather, aim for control of symptoms, employing topical care if possible.

BW

108

Lichen Sclerosis et Atrophicus

Kraurosis Vulvae • Balanitis Xerotica Obliterans

Patients can be divided into three clinical groups for management: prepubertal children, adults with genital disease, and adults with extragenital disease. Prepubertal children often have spontaneous clearing at menarche. Extragenital disease is often quite refractory to therapy, but is often asymptomatic. Aggressiveness of therapy is determined by the severity of the symptoms (usually burning or pruritus).

Initial Therapy

Testosterone propionate 2% ointment (compounded by mixing 30 ml testosterone propionate in oil with 120 g petroleum) is applied with gentle massage b.i.d. or t.i.d. Response may be quite slow, and a

6-month trial is required to establish efficacy. Therapy must be continued indefinitely, but may be decreased to as little as a once-weekly application. Men and postmenopausal women respond best.

Alternative Therapy

1. Topical steroids may help relieve pruritus, but must be used with caution in the genital area. A recent report of aggressive 3-month treatment with clobetasol propionate (Temovate) for genital lichen sclerosis et atrophicus (LS&A) showed good results.
2. Topical progesterone in oil 100 mg/oz of emollient (Aquaphor) applied b.i.d. may also be effective. Prepubertal children and premenopausal women are good candidates for this therapy.

Subsequent Therapy

The following systemic therapies are for those who have failed the above treatments.

1. Potassium P-aminobenzoate (Potaba) beginning at 12 g/day in divided doses has been reported to be successful for genital and extragenital LS&A. The dose may be increased to 24 g/day. For children, use 1 g/10 lbs. Response may require 8 weeks of therapy.
2. Hydroxychloroquine (Plaquenil) 200 mg q.d. or b.i.d. may be helpful. Regular ophthalmic examination is required.
3. Etretinate (Tegison) 1 mg/kg/day improved six of eight patients in an uncontrolled study. All patients experienced retinoid side effects (see Appendix 6).
4. Intractable pruritus may respond to injections of absolute alcohol 0.1 cc/cm^2 in the upper subcutaneous tissue. Sloughing of skin may occur, and response is variable.

Pitfalls

1. Laser and excisional surgery may be followed by recurrence, and should not be undertaken except by experts in this disease and should not be used except in those patients failing other forms of treatment. Vulvectomy is not indicated except for neoplasia.
2. Topical testosterone may lead to clitoral hypertrophy and an increase in libido. Older women may discontinue therapy for this reason.
3. For the side effects of the retinoids and topical steroids, see Appendices 6 and 3.

4. Potassium *p*-aminobenzoate (Potaba) therapy may lead to GI upset, rashes, hypoglycemia, leukopenia, and, rarely, hepatotoxicity. It is contraindicated in patients allergic to *p*-aminobenzoic acid and sulfonamides. Potassium *p*-aminobenzoate will interfere with the efficacy of sulfonamide antibiotics, so it must be stopped if an antibiotic of this class is used.
5. The side effects of hydroxychloroquine include retinal toxicity, rashes, and GI upset. Psoriasis may flare or become erythrodermic.

TB

109

Lichen Simplex Chronicus

Lichen simplex chronicus (LSC) identifies chronically pruritic plaque(s) that have been rubbed or excoriated to the point of epidermal hyperplasia and dermal fibrosis. Lesions of LSC may occur without other skin disease or may be a feature of any chronic pruritic dermatosis (e.g., atopic dermatitis or psoriasis). For treatment of an associated skin disease refer to the appropriate chapter. Lesions of LSC commonly occur on the ankles, elbows, or genital area.

Initial Therapy

1. Explain the role of rubbing or scratching to the patient.
2. Oral antihistamines (hydroxyzine or dipenhydramine) 25–50 mg q.h.s. and as tolerated during the day.
3. For nongenital areas apply a high-potency to superpotency steroid ointment b.i.d. for 2 weeks.
4. For genital lesions prescribe hydrocortisone 2.5% cream to be applied p.r.n. to control itching. Look for associated or underlying tinea cruris, pediculosis, and erythrasma.

Alternative Therapy

For very thick plaques triamcinolone acetonide (Kenalog) suspension (5–10 mg/cc) may be injected into the dermis of the lesion.

Subsequent Therapy

LESION(S) IMPROVED WITH INITIAL THERAPY
Reduce the strength of the topical steroid.

LESIONS UNIMPROVED WITH INITIAL THERAPY
1. Nongenital lesions
    a. Increase the frequency of application of the topical steroid *and* occlude the steroid at night.
    b. Cover the lesion 24 hours a day to prevent scratching. Cordran tape, a permeable dressing (Duoderm), or simple plastic wrap may be used.
    c. Add a topical tar preparation to the topical steroid. *Do not occlude.*
    d. Inject triamcinolone acetonide suspension (5–10 mg/cc) into the dermis of the lesion biweekly until it clears.
2. Genital lesions
    a. Apply a stronger nonfluorinated steroid and praxomine cream (PRAX) t.i.d.
    b. Apply an imidazole cream b.i.d. with the nonfluorinated steroid and praxomine cream.
    c. Iodochlorhydroxyquin-hydrocortisone (Vioform HC) may aid an occasional patient. However, it can stain the underclothing yellow.
3. Occasional patients with totally refractory LSC may have an underlying psychological disorder that may require adjunctive psychotherapy.

Pitfalls

1. The application of steroids to the genital area may lead to rebound pruritus when they are stopped. In addition striae and atrophy are common complications. Use caution when applying topical steroids in this area.
2. Intralesional steroid injections may be associated with local atrophy and occasionally atrophy, alopecia, and hypopigmentation along draining lymphatic channels. See Appendix 4.

TB

110

Linear IgA Dermatosis

Linear IgA dermatosis is a bullous disorder that resembles dermatitis herpetiformis but is distinguished from this disorder by the linear deposition of IgA at the epidermodermal junction and the absence of gluten-sensitive enteropathy. The therapeutic goal is control of blister formation.

Initial Therapy

Linear IgA dermatosis is initially treated with oral dapsone 100 mg/day. Expect a clinical response within 5–10 days. If blistering is not controlled, increase dapsone every 1–2 weeks in 100-mg increments until the desired clinical response is obtained. Most patients will require 300 mg or less. If control is not achieved, dapsone may be gradually increased if clinically significant hemolysis or methemoglobinemia are not encountered. Check CBC weekly or every 2 weeks as dapsone is increased.

Subsequent Therapy

Taper dapsone by 50-mg increments every 2 weeks until the appropriate maintenance dose is achieved. The maintenance dose should be the level at which the patient gets an occasional blister. Continue therapy indefinitely.

Alternative Therapy

1. Sulfapyridine offers an alternative for dapsone-allergic individuals or for patients who do not tolerate its side effects of nausea, lethargy, and depression. Use an initial dose of 500 mg b.i.d. and increase dose by 1 g every 1–2 weeks until the disease is controlled. Control may require 1–4 g/day.
2. If partial control is attained with maximal doses of sulfapyridine (4 g/day), benefit may be derived by adding small amounts of dapsone (25–50 mg/day).

Pitfalls

1. Patients should be screened for G6PD deficiency, as dapsone causes acute hemolysis in these individiuals. However, under extremely unusual circumstances (no other alternatives), dapsone may be used in such individuals, but should be started at low doses (25–50 mg/day). After hemolysis, the dose can be raised, but chronic hemolysis must be balanced against therapeutic benefit.
2. Monitor hemoglobin and hematocrit, as dapsone causes dose-related hemolysis and methemoglobinemia.
3. Although a rare complication, dapsone causes hepatitis and renal toxicity (see Ch. 84, Hansen's disease).
4. If the patient does not respond to dapsone or sulfapyridine, the diagnosis should be reevaluated.

BW

111

Linear Scleroderma

Linear Morphea • En Coup de Sabre

Linear scleroderma is a form of localized sclerosis most common in children or adolescents that can be progressive, leading to severe disability and disfigurement. Linear scleroderma tends to involute spontaneously less than morphea. Linear scleroderma also may be related to hemiatrophy syndromes such as Romberg's disease.

Initial Therapy

1. Phenytoin sodium (Dilantin) 100 mg b.i.d. or t.i.d., depending on age and body weight, may produce softening of sclerotic skin within 2–4 months, and substantial clearing within 1–2 years.
2. Physical therapy, involving both active and passive stretching exercises, is necessary to prevent contractures.

Alternative Therapy

1. Either chemotherapeutic agents or penicillamine can be tried for progressive cases not responding to phenytoin (see Ch. 157).
2. Surgery may be needed for severe contractures that do not respond to physical therapy.

Subsequent Therapy

1. Cosmetically disfiguring lesions can be treated with intralesional bovine collagen (Zyplast). *Note:* Skin testing is required to rule out allergy (5%–10% of the population may be allergic).
2. Alternative cosmetic therapy: Liquid silicone or fat implants and/or lipoinjection also have been used to improve cosmetic deformities on the face. *Note:* Cosmetic correction should be performed only by those who are expert in the application of these materials.

Pitfalls

1. Because phenytoin impairs vitamin D metabolism in the liver, osteomalacia or rickets can occur during long-term therapy; patients undergoing long-term therapy should also receive oral vitamin D (400 U/day). Numerous important drug interactions and potential side effects occur with phenytoin (see Ch. 54, Epidermolysis Bullosa).
2. The side effects of chemotherapeutic agents and penicillamine are discussed in Appendix 7 and Ch. 157, Systemic Scleroderma, respectively.

PE

112

Lipoma

Lipomas are benign, and their therapy is for cosmesis only. If they contain a significant vascular component (angiolipoma), they may be tender. All therapies are surgical.

Initial Therapy

After administration of local anesthesia, a 4–6-mm cylinder of skin is removed over the center of the lipoma. A medium-sized curette is used to break up the lipoma, and the contents are extruded through the small hole. The hole is sutured, and a pressure dressing applied. A large lipoma may be extracted through a small hole with minimal scarring.

Alternative Therapy

1. Standard surgical excision gives excellent results, but often leaves a substantial scar.
2. Liposuction may be used to remove very large (greater than 5 cm) lipomas through smaller defects.

Pitfalls

1. Lipomas over the midline (spine) may be associated with or continuous with a defect or lipoma of the spinal canal. These lesions should only be approached by neurosurgeons. A CT scan or MRI is an essential part of their preoperative evaluation.
2. Epidermal inclusion cysts must be differentiated from lipomas.

TB

113

Localized Scleroderma

Morphea

The prognosis for patients with localized scleroderma is guardedly optimistic: many cases disappear spontaneously, and most are limited to small inconsequential areas. Therefore, aggressive therapy should be administered only to patients with widespread or rapidly advancing disease.

Initial Therapy

1. Prescribe a superpotent topical steroid cream (see Appendix 1) to be applied over areas of active inflammation (lilac or red surrounding ring).
2. Intralesional triamcinolone acetonide (Kenalog) 5 mg/cc may slow progression if injected into the margin of lesions.

Alternative Therapy

1. Several reports suggest that sulfasalazine (Azulfidine) 1 g b.i.d. can abort or reverse morphea. Therapy must be continued for at least 4 months.
2. Phenytoin sodium (Dilantin) 100 mg b.i.d. increasing as needed to 100 mg q.i.d. has been helpful in some cases of localized scleroderma. *Note:* Blood levels must be monitored to ensure adequate dosing.
3. Chemotherapeutic agents or penicillamine (see Ch. 157, Systemic Scleroderma) can be used for severe, progressive disease unresponsive to the above regimen. Systemic steroids are of no help.

Ancillary Therapy

1. Trauma should be avoided.
2. Daily lubrication is beneficial.
3. Passive and active physical therapy may prevent contractures when lesions overlie joints.

Pitfalls

1. The pitfalls of topical steroids are described in Appendix 3.
2. The side effects and drug interactions of phenytoin are protean (see Chs. 54 and 111).
3. Sulfasalazine is associated with a high frequency of hematologic, GI, and cutaneous side effects with which the physician must be familiar before prescribing this drug. Oligospermia can occur in males. A screen for possible G6DP deficiency is required before initiating therapy.

PE

114

Lymphocytoma Cutis/Lymphoid Hyperplasia

Included in this disease group are lesions attributable to drugs (e.g., diphenylhydantoin), insect bites, spirochetes (*B. burgdorferi*), and early undiagnosable lymphoid malignancies. Differentiating these entities by means of routine histology may be extremely difficult. In those cases in which the diagnosis is unclear, studies should be undertaken to determine whether the infiltrate is monoclonal or polyclonal. Monoclonal cases should be considered as possibly malignant. In borderline cases a complete evaluation to exclude systemic lymphoma should be considered.

Initial Therapy

1. Stop possible incriminating drugs, and question about insect or arachnid bites (especially those of ticks). The value of serologic tests for *B. burgdorferi* in this setting is unknown, but antibodies to the spirochete have been detected in European cases. This presentation of Lyme disease appears to be rare or unrecognized in the United States.
2. If the lesion is solitary and easily removed, total surgical excision may be curative. A portion of the excised lesion should be frozen to provide adequate material for special studies (e.g. gene rearrangements).
3. In cases where *B. burgdorferi* is a possible precipitating cause (especially earlobe lesions), an empiric trial of penicillin V, or in penicillin-allergic patients, tetracycline 500 mg q.i.d., for 10 days may be of benefit.
4. Application of intermediate- to high-potency steroids with occlusion will occasionally clear lesions. If this fails, a trial with a superpotent steroid may be effective.
5. Intralesional corticosteroids (triamcinalone acetonide 5–10 mg/cc) will significantly reduce or eliminate lesions.

Alternative Therapy

Superficial radiation therapy is almost always effective.

Subsequent Therapy

Regular follow-up is essential, as cases of malignant lymphoma have initially been diagnosed as benign.

Pitfalls

1. In all cases in which there is no clear precipitating cause, the possibility of malignancy must be entertained. Special studies, consultation, and/or referral should be considered.
2. For side effects of topical and intralesional steroids, see Appendices 3 and 4.
3. Local atrophy, telangiectasia, and malignancies may occur following radiation therapy. Radiation therapy is contraindicated in pregnancy.

TB

115

Lymphogranuloma Venereum

Initial Therapy

Treat with oral tetracycline 500 mg q.i.d. for at least 3 weeks.

Alternative Therapy

1. Sulfisoxazole 4 g initially and 500 mg q.i.d. for at least 3 weeks.
2. Minocycline 100 mg b.i.d. for at least 3 weeks.
3. Oral erythromycin 500 mg q.i.d. for at least 3 weeks.

Subsequent Therapy

1. Fluctuant nodes should be aspirated, not incised and drained.
2. Rectal stricture may be managed by recurrent dilatation.

Pitfalls

1. Sometimes multiple courses of antibiotics are required.
2. Surgical excision of lymph nodes or extensive lymphedematous areas is contraindicated, as it may worsen lymphedema.
3. Surgery should not be performed during active phases of the disease, and when performed, should be preceded and followed by 2 weeks of antibiotic treatment.

TB

116

Malignant Melanoma

The therapy of malignant melanoma is directed by the thickness of the lesion and its Clark's level. Therapy is largely surgical. Only treatment of primary lesions is discussed. Although occasional patients with local recurrence or metastasis may be salvaged by additional surgical or chemotherapeutic procedures, the primary focus must be to adequately excise the lesion at the time of initial definitive diagnosis.

Two areas of considerable controversy are:

1. What constitutes adequate margins of resection of the primary tumor?
2. Which patients should have elective regional lymph node dissection? In questionable cases, referral to regional centers or consultation with regional experts is recommended.

Initial Therapy

1. For diagnosis, an in toto excisional biopsy with minimal margins, pathologically evaluated at multiple levels to determine the maximum depth, is highly recommended. For large lesions that cannot be excised without a major surgical procedure or significant cosmetic deformity, an incisional biopsy of the clinically thickest-appearing area is permissible.
2. For malignant melanoma in situ, and for lesions less than 1 mm thick

(Clark's level III or less), an excision of 1 cm of normal skin is considered adequate.

3. For malignant melanomas greater than 1 mm thick, a normal skin margin of 3 cm is adequate. (For lesions 1–2 mm thick, one large series supports a 1-cm margin, although follow-up is too short to absolutely recommend this reduced skin margin.)

4. Obtain a baseline history, physical examination (especially noting any enlarged lymph nodes), a CBC, a multipanel chemistry profile, and a chest x-ray for all patients.

5. Patients with higher-risk lesions (over 1 mm thick or Clark's level III or more) may be considered for more extensive base-line tests searching for metastases (CT of the brain, chest, or abdomen), especially if regional lymph node dissection is considered.

Ancillary Therapy

1. Elective regional lymph node dissection of clinically negative nodes is *not* indicated for patients with primary lesions of 1 mm or less in thickness, as regional lymph node recurrence is rare.

2. Elective regional lymph node dissection of clinically negative nodes is also *not* indicated for patients with primary lesions at least 4 mm thick, as widespread recurrence is common and not affected by regional lymph node dissection.

3. Advanced age or illness (where death from another disease is likely) is a relative contraindication to elective lymph node dissection.

4. If the draining lymph node group cannot be determined (i.e., midline lesions, trunk lesions), elective regional lymph node dissection is not indicated. Technetium lymphoscintigraphy may help to determine the draining group.

5. Consider for elective lymph node dissection any patients with lesions of intermediate thickness (1–4 mm and level IV lesions over 0.76 mm) with no evidence of distant metastases.

6. Remove clinically involved nodes to obtain local control.

Pitfalls

1. Failure to biopsy a suspicious lesion is the most serious pitfall.

2. An inadequate initial biopsy or pathologic evaluation is a major pitfall that may result in inadequate therapy. An *excisional* biopsy is highly recommended. The pathology report must include the thickness and Clark's level.

3. Melanoma is unpredictable. Remain constantly suspicious of the possibility of metastasis or recurrence.

4. Seek consultation in all but the most straightforward cases both in pathologic diagnosis and current therapy. Refer to regional centers.

Subsequent Therapy

Follow patients at 3-month intervals during the first year, then at 6-month intervals thereafter. Regular radiographic and laboratory examinations are indicated for patients with intermediate- and high-risk lesions (1.5 mm or greater, and Clark's level IV over 0.76 mm).

TB

117

Mastocytosis

Uticaria Pigmentosa

Therapy attempts to control symptoms of *localized* or *systemic* mastocytosis. Symptoms result from release of mast cell mediators, and therapy must therefore be tailored to each patient's clinical state.

LOCALIZED MASTOCYTOSIS

Children with localized mast cell tumors are best treated by parental reassurance. Most lesions slowly resolve spontaneously. In an occasional symptomatic case, excision of the lesion may be appropriate. Because superpotent steroids cause mast cells to disappear from skin, the q.d. application of these agents to mast cell tumors for 4–6 weeks seems reasonable.

SYSTEMIC MASTOCYTOSIS

Symptoms caused by systemic mastocytosis include pruritus and whealing, episodic hypotension and flushing, GI symptoms, and bothersome cutaneous lesions.

Initial Therapy

PATIENTS WITH PRURITUS AND WHEALING

1. Treat with oral H_1 antihistamine to maintain pharmacologic action 24 h/day. Oral hydroxyzine (Atarax) 25–50 mg q.i.d. for adults and 1–2 tsp t.i.d. in children is excellent, but frequently causes sedation. Terfenidine (Seldane) 60–120 mg b.i.d., or astemizole (Hismanal) 10–20 mg/day, may be efficacious and do not usually cause sedation.
2. Avoid symptom-causing agents, including aspirin, NSAIDs, morphine, iodine, d-tubocurarine, polymixins, and decamethonium. Advise the patient to avoid alcohol if exacerbation of symptoms is observed.

PATIENTS WITH EPISODIC HYPOTENSION AND FLUSHING

1. These patients usually do not respond to H_1 and H_2 blockers alone, although aspirin and NSAIDS may be useful. Since NSAIDS may cause mast cell histamine release, give H_1 and H_2 antihistamines concomitantly (e.g., hydroxyzine 25–50 mg q.i.d., plus 300 mg cimetidine q.i.d.).
2. After 3–4 days, give aspirin 640–975 mg q.i.d. and attempt to achieve salicylate levels of 20–30 mg/ml. Naproxen (e.g., Naprosyn) 375 mg b.i.d. or ibuprofen (e.g., Motrin) 600 mg b.i.d. may also be used. Because aspirin may induce hypotension and flushing even in this setting, it is best to initiate aspirin therapy in a hospital setting.

PATIENTS WITH GASTROINTESTINAL SYMPTOMS

Oral administration of disodium cromoglycate (adult dosage 100–200 mg q.i.d.) is useful.

PATIENTS WITH BOTHERSOME CUTANEOUS LESIONS

Potent fluorinated steroids cause disappearance of mast cells from the skin. Prescribe a superpotent steroid cream (Diprolene or Temovate) to be applied under occlusion for 6 hours for 6 weeks. The skin will remain clear for the following year, and can be retreated as necessary.

Subsequent Therapy

PATIENTS WITH PRURITUS AND WHEALING

1. Reduce or maintain antihistamine at the dose necessary to control the patient's symptoms, and maintain therapy indefinitely.

2. If adequate control of symptoms is not possible, add an H_2 antagonist (e.g., cimetidine 400 mg q.i.d.).

Alternative Therapy

PATIENTS WITH PRURITUS AND WHEALING

1. Oral disodium cromoglycate (adult dose: 100–200 mg q.i.d., up to 40 mg/kg) may be useful despite poor absorption. Tablets for inhalation may be taken orally or dissolved in water.
2. Phototherapy (PUVA) may be useful. Treat patients 2–4 ×/week until dermographism is relieved. Remission may last up to 10 months.

BW

118

Miliaria

Of the three types of miliaria (crystallina, rubra, and profunda), profunda is only rarely seen in a nonmilitary setting. Both miliaria rubra and miliaria profunda can cause abnormal sweat gland function, leading potentially to varying degrees of heat intolerance owing to interference with normal evaporative water loss.

Initial Therapy

1. Cool the environment; allow air to circulate, and turn the patient frequently enough to minimize sweating and occlusion.
2. Control fever if it is part of another systemic illness.
3. Application of a medium-potency topical steroid cream (e.g., triamcinolone acetonide 0.1% (Kenalog) or fluocinolone 0.1% (Synalar) b.i.d.) will minimize the itch, and the lanolin-containing cream vehicles may themselves be beneficial for miliaria.
4. A camphor-menthol-phenol-containing lotion (e.g., Sarna) can be employed to relieve itching.
5. Antihistamines, such as oral hydroxyzine (Atarax) 10–25 mg t.i.d., may be

helpful for itch. Oral terfenidine (Seldane) 60 mg b.i.d. is a less soporific, but somewhat less effective (and more expensive), alternative.

Subsequent Therapy

1. Although the rash should respond quickly to the above measures, sweat gland dysfunction of involved areas will be present for up to 2 weeks after episodes of miliaria rubra (longer for miliaria profunda; no sweat gland dysfunction is associated with miliaria crystallina). Patients with extensive miliaria, therefore, may be at risk for heat intolerance and should be warned to avoid excessive exercise.
2. Ascorbic acid (1–2 g/day), in uncontrolled studies, has been reported to prevent recurrences of miliaria in those at risk.

Pitfalls

1. Recognition is critical because a superficial folliculitis can occur under the same conditions (i.e., occlusion, fever, sluggish air movement). The presence of follicular pustules allows this distinction to be made.
2. Heat stroke, as a result of sweat gland dysfunction, is a rare complication of miliaria.
3. Development of kidney stones has been reported in patients taking high doses of ascorbic acid. This may be exacerbated by dehydration.

PE

119

Molluscum Contagiosum

The therapy of molluscum contagiosum is divided into three treatment groups: children, adults, and the immunosuppressed. Molluscum contagiosum limited to the genital area in children should raise the possibility of child abuse.

CHILDREN

Children may have a few lesions or many lesions (50 to hundreds).

Initial Therapy

OVER 50 LESIONS
For children with many lesions no therapy should be attempted. These lesions will eventually spontaneously disappear without sequelae. Parents are reluctant to accept this option, but heroic measures are unnecessary and potentially scarring both physically and emotionally.

UNDER 50 LESIONS
If the number of lesions is manageable and the child is at least in part cooperative, multiple topical therapies may work.

1. Administer cryotherapy with liquid nitrogen to the individual lesions.
2. Apply 1 *tiny* drop of cantharidin to the tip of each lesion and wash off in 2–6 hours. Do not occlude. Before allowing the patient to move around, be sure the medication is dry to the touch so it does not spread to normal skin. Lesions will crust and fall off in less than 1 week. This medication must be applied by the doctor in the office. It cannot be used in occluded areas (axillae, groin, inner thighs) or around the eyes.
3. Pricking the surface of a lesion with a #11 blade will often lead to inflammation and resolution of that lesion. Pressing out the central core with a comedone extractor will guarantee resolution of that lesion.
4. Cooperative children may occasionally be able to tolerate the pain of curetting individual lesions.

ADULTS

Molluscum contagiosum in nonimmunosuppressed adults is usually an STD, and is found in the genital area. Adults with extensive lesions outside the genital area must be evaluated for immunosuppression, especially HIV infection.

Initial Therapy

1. Cryotherapy with liquid nitrogen is quick and effective.
2. Evaluate for other STDs.
3. Examine and treat the patient's sexual partner(s).
4. Advise the patient that the lesions are sexually transmissable.

Alternative Therapy

1. Destruction of each lesion by pricking with a large (18-guage) needle or a #11 blade. Removal of the core with a comedone extractor will enhance resolution.
2. Adults will usually tolerate curettage of individual lesions.

Subsequent Therapy

One treatment is usually inadequate to eradicate all lesions. See the patient at biweekly intervals until no lesions are present, then 4–6 weeks after the last visit for a final check.

Pitfalls

1. The most common error is diagnosing molluscum as genital warts. If there is any question, refer the patient.
2. Avoid cantharidin in the genital area.

IMMUNOSUPPRESSED

In severe immunosuppression, especially in ARC or AIDS, extensive facial or genital molluscum are very common. Total cure is almost impossible. (Individual lesions in general do not spontaneously resolve as in healthy adults and children.) Lesions are treated for cosmesis at the patient's request.

Initial Therapy

1. Liquid nitrogen cryotherapy (preferably by spray rather than a swab) is effective and well tolerated.
2. For facial or truncal molluscum, cantharidin applied for 2–6 hours and then washed off will also resolve lesions. This has the advantage of usually being painless.
3. Instruct the patient to use only an electric razor (preferably with floating heads) to shave. This type of shaving is less likely to spread the lesions.

Alternative Therapy

Pricking and curetting lesions, although also effective, have disadvantages: First, they are potentially hazardous to the care provider because he may be exposed to blood. Second, they may provide a portal of entry for infection. If these methods are used, appropriate precautions are necessary.

Pitfall

In the setting of immunosuppression, other infectious agents (e.g., herpes simplex, cryptococcus neoformans) may produce lesions mimicking molluscum contagiosum. If there is any question as to the correct diagnosis, a biopsy is indicated.

TB

120

Mucha-Habermann Disease

Pityriasis Lichenoides et Variolaformis Acuta • Pityriasis Lichenoides Chronica • Lymphomatoid Papulosis

These closely related lymphocytic angiitides had been considered benign. About 10% of reported cases of lymphomatoid papulosis (LYP) have been associated with lymphoreticular malignancy, supporting the concept that LYP may be a premalignant process. Whether aggressive therapy will alter progression to malignancy is unknown. Pityriasis lichenoides chronica (PLC) is treated like pityriasis lichenoides et variolaformis acuta (PLEVA).

Initial Therapy

1. Oral antibiotics, usually tetracycline or erythromycin 250 mg to 500 mg q.i.d.
2. Mild PLC and PLEVA may be treated with intermediate-strength topical steroids if few lesions are present.

Alternative Therapy

UVB phototherapy with natural sunlight or a home or office light box is usually quite effective, especially in PLEVA and PLC.

Subsequent Therapy

Most patients are managed with the above modalities. Exceptional patients with progressive or incapacitating disease may be considered for the following therapies:

1. Photochemotherapy (PUVA) (psoralens plus UVA) may clear PLEVA, PLC, and LYP, and usually requires doses lower than required for psoriasis. Some patients may require maintenance therapy.
2. Low-dose oral methotrexate 7.5–20 mg/week is usually quite efficacious. Recurrences may occur.
3. Topical carmustine (BCNU) 10 mg/60 ml q.d. has been used to treat LYP. Therapy did not lead to remission.

Pitfalls

1. Tetracycline is contraindicated in pregnancy and in children under 8 years of age.
2. Because PLEVA and PLC are benign disorders, PUVA and methotrexate should be reserved for severe cases, and informed consent is essential.
3. For complications of PUVA and methotrexate therapy see Ch. 147, Psoriasis.
4. Lymphomatoid papulosis and PLEVA may appear clinically similar. A biopsy of one or more lesions is necessary to establish the correct diagnosis.

TB

121

Mucocutaneous Lymph Node Syndrome

Kawasaki Disease

Mucocutaneous lymph node syndrome (MCLS) is an acute, febrile disease of infants and young children. About one-third of patients develop coronary arterial sequelae, including aneurysms. No specific therapy is available.

Initial Therapy

1. Recent studies (See Pediatrics 82:122, 1988) suggest that gamma globulin 400 mg/kg/day for 4 successive days, administered by intravenous infusion over 1–2 hours, as early as possible in the course of the disease (within 10 days of onset), may prevent the coronary sequelae of the disease.
2. Administer aspirin, at doses of 80–100 mg/kg/day, for both its antiinflammatory and its anticoagulant properties, for a total of 8 weeks and then reduce the dosage to 30 mg/kg/day for 2 months after the fever has subsided.
3. Manage cardiac complications by consultation with a pediatric cardiologist.
4. Perform a work-up for MCLS, including WBC, ESR, C-reactive protein, protein electrophoresis (-2 globulin is increased in MCLS), platelet counts, ASLO titers to rule out poststreptococcal rheumatic fever, and both electro- and echocardiogram. Follow ESR and C-reactive protein levels at weekly intervals to assess disease activity. Perform angiography in patients whose fever persists for more than 15 days, in cases where febrile episodes recur and in cases in which both ESR and C-reactive protein remain elevated for over 1 month.

Ancillary Therapy

Antibiotics can be discontinued after the diagnosis is established.

Pitfalls

1. The cardiac sequelae of MCLS represent the major complication of this disease.
2. Avoid systemic steroids; prior studies suggest a worse prognosis in steroid-treated cases.
3. Serum salicylate levels should be monitored in patients receiving high dosages of aspirin.

PE

122

Myiasis

Myiasis is caused by the larvae of certain botfly species that develop in the skin. In addition to direct inoculation by the fly, the larvae may enter the skin from the bites of other insects who carry the botfly eggs, or by direct skin contact with the eggs deposited on beaches or clothing. Most cases are acquired in the tropics of Central and South America and Africa, but cases have been acquired in most areas of the United States.

Initial Therapy

1. Early recognition is important. A firm papule with a serous central discharge and a central orifice should suggest the diagnosis.
2. Occasionally, gentle pressure laterally will express the larva.
3. If this fails, anesthetize the lesion, incise the skin adjacent to the larva, and remove it with a hemostat or curette.

Ancillary Therapy

1. Secondary infection is very common and should be treated if present.
2. Pruritus and swelling at the site may occur owing to an allergic reaction to the larvae. Oral hydroxyzine or diphenhydramine 25–50 mg q.h.s. and t.i.d. may benefit.

TB

123

Necrobiosis Lipoidica Diabeticorum

Lesions of necrobiosis lipoidica diabeticorum (NLD) are usually, but not always, associated with juvenile-onset diabetes. Tending to occur singly or in crops on the anterior lower legs, they can, however, appear anywhere on the body. Lesions on the leg exhibit more of a tendency to ulcerate than lesions elsewhere.

Initial Therapy

1. For nonulcerated, symptomatic lesions (asymptomatic lesions need not be treated), intralesional triamcinolone acetonide (10-mg/ml stock solution is diluted 1:2 with normal saline or lidocaine (final concentration: approximately 3 mg/cc)). Small amounts of this solution are injected intradermally into plaques via a 30-guage needle. Injections then are repeated every 2–3 weeks.
2. Ulcers present in lesions of NLD need to heal prior to steroid administration. Wound healing with standard wet-to-dry dressings and antibiotic creams can be very slow, especially in insulin-dependent diabetics. Therefore, vapor-permeable membranes (e.g., Op-Site, Duoderm, or Tegaderm) should be applied over individual ulcers, and changed weekly until healing of the ulcer has occurred.

Alternate Therapy

1. A combination of dipyridimole (Persantine) and aspirin has been reported to benefit some patients with NLD.
2. Administration of pentoxiphylline (Trental) 400 mg t.i.d. for 3–4 weeks has been reported to benefit some patients with NLD.
3. Applications of a superpotent topical steroid (see Appendix 1) will occasionally produce some reduction in lesion size and symptoms.

Subsequent Therapy

1. After ulcers are healed, intralesional steroids can be administered, as described above.

2. Elevation and compression stockings reduce associated lymphedema and may both hasten healing and prevent new episodes of ulceration.
3. If the patient has not yet been evaluated for diabetes, a work-up is in order.

Pitfalls

1. Lesions of NLD can be very resistant to the above management, and may not respond. Moreover, new lesions may continue to form.
2. There is no relationship between severity of NLD and diabetic status.

PE

124

Necrolytic Migratory Erythema

Glucagonoma Syndrome

Necrolytic migratory erythema (NME) occurs almost exclusively in patients with underlying glucagon-secreting tumors of the pancreas. By the time of diagnosis, most patients already demonstrate hepatic metastases.

Initial Therapy

1. Work-up for a glucagon-secreting tumor, including serum glucagon, fasting blood glucose, serum amino acids (if available), protein levels, and celiac angiography, is mandatory.
2. A skin biopsy is useful in differentiating NME from other eczematous, intertriginous eruptions (see Pitfalls).
3. If a primary tumor is found prior to hepatic metastases, excision is usually curative.
4. Chemotherapy, under the supervision of a hematologist-oncologist, is helpful in metastatic cases. Both streptozotocin and 5-(3,3-dimethyl-1-troazemo) imidazole carboxyamide (DTIC) reportedly are effective.

Ancillary Therapy

1. Amino acid infusion may help the dermatitis, as well as the systemic consequences of hypoaminoacidemia, even in the face of unresectable tumors.
2. A potent topical steroid is useful for the dermatitis (give low-potency, nonfluorinated preparations for facial or intertriginous lesions) (see Appendix 1).

Pitfalls

1. A rash virtually identical to NME can occur in a number of other clinical settings, including acrodermatitis enteropathica, histiocytosis- X, certain inherited disorders of amino acid metabolism, and essential fatty acid deficiency. These diagnostic possibilities should be considered in the work-up of patients with NME-like rashes.
2. Plasma glucagon is not a routint test; check with the laboratory for instructions in mode of collection (e.g., addition of a proteinase inhibitor).
3. Streptozotocin administration is often accompanied by nausea, and both renal and hepatic toxicity may occur.
4. Bone marrow toxicity is the most important side effect of DTIC therapy.

PE

125

Neurotic Excoriation

Neurotic excoriation describes various forms of psychogenic excoriations seen in dermatologic practice. Although it implies neurosis as the cause, the exact nature of the underlying psychopathology may range from anxiety disorder, including obsessive-compulsive disorders, to major depressive episodes. Consequently, the therapeutic approach varies depending on the nature of the underlying psychopathology involved. *Correct diagnosis* of underlying psychopathology is critical in selecting appropriate therapy.

The goal of therapy is twofold: to treat the underlying psychopathology and to prevent secondary complications such as cellulitis and osteomyelitis resulting from deep excoriations. The following outline constitutes a reasonable and practical approach.

Initial Therapy

1. Obtain consultation from a mental health professional to ascertain diagnosis and initiate psychotherapy if indicated.
2. If the patient resists psychiatric referral, treatment with psychopharmacologic agents may be considered. Excoriators with significant underlying depression may benefit from the oral tricyclic antidepressant doxepin 25 mg q.h.s., increasing by 25 mg every 3–7 days as tolerated until therapeutic dose of 100 mg to as much as 300 mg q.h.s. is reached. Doxepin also has significant antipruritic and antianxiety effects. Side effects include sedation, orthostatic hypotension, anticholinergic effects such as constipation, and cardiac side effects such as prolongation of Q-T interval. Check doxepin blood level if significant low-dose side effects occur or if there is no response at high doses. The therapeutic level of doxepin is between 100 and 200 μg/L of the sum of doxepin and its metabolite nordoxepin.
3. Excoriators with anxiety disorder can be treated with an antianxiety agent such as oral alprazolam (Xanax) 0.25–0.5 mg q.i.d. p.r.n.; the main side effect is sedation. Long-term use of alprazolam may cause addiction. Alternatively, a nonsedating antianxiety agent such as oral buspirone (BuSpar) 5 mg t.i.d. can be initiated, gradually increasing the dose until the desired effect is obtained. Onset of therapeutic efficacy of buspirone is often delayed as much as 2–3 weeks, however, and therefore buspirone can not be used on a p.r.n. basis. Buspirone is nonaddictive.
4. Patients with obsessive-compulsive tendencies are frequently treated successfully with a behavioral therapy regimen. Medications with anticompulsive activity (e.g., clomipramine) have not been released in the United States, and the use of fluoxetine hydrochloride (Prozac) for treatment of obsessive-compulsive disorders has not yet been approved by the FDA, although fluoxetine hydrochloride is available for treatment of depression.
5. Secondary complications of excoriations may need to be treated with topical or systemic antibiotics. If severe pain results from deep excoriation, occlusive dressings (e.g., Duoderm) may control the pain, facilitate healing, and prevent further excoriation.

Alternative Therapy

For patients not responding to the above therapy or who cannot receive the above therapy owing to complicating factors:

1. If doxepin is contraindicated (e.g., cardiac arrythmia, severe constipation), try trazodone or fluoxetine hydrochloride.
2. If the agitated subtype of depression is present, prescribe a benzodiazapine with antidepressant activity (e.g., alprazolam).
3. If sedative side effects of doxepin occur, prescribe a less sedating tricyclic antidepressant (e.g., desipramine) along with a traditional antihistamine such as hydroxyzine.
4. If the patient presents with delusional symptoms and excoriations, primary therapy may include the use of antipsychotic agents with or without an antidepressant. Refer to Chapter 42, Delusions of Parasitosis (formication) for information regarding the use of antipsychotic agents.

BW

126

Nevus Sebaceus

Organoid Nevus

This isolated hamartoma presents early in life as an atrophic yellow patch on the vertex or occiput of the scalp. During puberty the lesion will become papillated.

Initial Therapy

1. Associated neurologic, ophthalmic, and musculoskeletal abnormalities (nevus sebaceus syndrome) may occur, usually with large lesions overlying the scalp.
2. Biopsy any papules or nodules that develop in a nevus sebaceus.

Subsequent Therapy

Because basal cell carcinomas and other adnexal tumors (benign and malignant) commonly develop in nevus sebaceus, give consideration to total removal of the lesion in early adulthood.

TB

127

Oral Hairy Leukoplakia

Oral hairy leukoplakia (OHL) has to date been pathognomonic of infection with the HIV virus. Therapy will clear but will not cure lesions, and OHL will usually reappear once treatment is stopped. Therapy is rarely indicated, as OHL is asymptomatic.

Initial Therapy

1. Patients with OHL must be evaluated for the presence of HIV infection, and a determination of the extent of immunosuppression must be made.
2. Treat the frequently associated thrush, if present, with oral nystatin suspension or clotrimazole troches.
3. Topical retinoic acid 0.1% cream applied b.i.d., or
4. Topical acyclovir (Zovirax) ointment applied to the lesion q.i.d.

Alternative Therapy

1. Oral acyclovir 2.0–3.2 g/day (400 mg 5x/day, or 800 mg q.i.d.) for 10–14 days.
2. OHL will resolve with intravenous acyclovir, but this is rarely indicated.
3. Patients failing on acyclovir may clear with 9-(1,3-dihydroxy-2-propoxymethyl guainine (DHPG), used for treatment of cytomegalovirus-induced disease (retinitis, colitis). DHPG is potentially toxic and is not indicated for treating OHL alone. If the patient is receiving this agent for cytomegalovirus-induced disease, the OHL may clear.

Subsequent Therapy

Chronic suppression with retinoic acid or topical oral acyclovir may be used. However, as OHL is totally asymptomatic and hidden, suppressive therapy has no proven benefit.

Pitfalls

1. Failure to evaluate for HIV infection.
2. Side effects from oral acyclovir are rare. They include rashes and mild GI

upset. Intravenous acyclovir may precipitate in the kidney and decrease renal function, so renal function tests should be followed.

3. HIV-positive individuals also may develop true precancerous or cancerous leukoplakic oral lesions. The diagnosis of OHL should be considered only when in its characteristic location (lateral tongue bilaterally). A biopsy is required to establish the diagnosis of OHL when seen at other locations in the oral cavity.

4. OHL is a clinical diagnosis. Epstein–Barr virus serologies play no role in the management or diagnosis of OHL.

TB

128

Palmoplantar Keratodermas

Palmoplantar keratodermas (PPK) can occur as a primary, inherited disorder of the volar surfaces, or as part of a generalized disorder, such as psoriasis, cutaneous T-cell lymphoma, or ichthyosis. Discussion of treatment here is limited to inherited forms only (see Ch. 147, Psoriasis, for management of volar lesions in that disease).

Initial Therapy

There is no uniformly effective therapy for PPK, but try all, alone or in combination, before administering systemic therapy. Reserve systemic therapy, particularly with oral retinoids, for incapacitated individuals.

1. Cracks and fissures: Application of flexible collodion 5% in ethyl acetate q.d. or b.i.d. This preparation burns upon application, but provides a protective film that may protect for several hours.

2. Salicylic acid 6% in propylene glycol 40% (Keralyt Gel) applied q.i.d. after bathing, or benzoic acid 3% in aquaphor ($\frac{1}{2}$-strength Whitfield's ointment) applied q.d. after bathing.

Alternative Therapy

1. If flexible colloidion is not helpful, tincture of benzoin (20–25%) in zinc oxide paste may be helpful.
2. If no improvement occurs, and the keratoderma interferes with either work or ambulation, the patient may be a candidate for oral retinoids. Currently, etretinate appears to be more effective than isotretinoin, but relatively high doses are usually required (e.g., 25 mg t.i.d. or q.i.d.). After 6 weeks, therapy should be adjusted upward or downward according to the initial response. *Note:* Systemic retinoids should be administered by physicians who have experience with the administration and side effects of these agents.

Subsequent Therapy

1. If some degree of relief is obtained with any of the above regimens, therapy should be continued on an indefinite basis, as these diseases are generally nonremitting.
2. The pitfalls of synthetic retinoids are discussed Appendix 1.
3. Some patients with PPK, treated with retinoids, develop severe skin fragility, which can make the patient more uncomfortable than prior to treatment, even in the face of substantial improvement of the PPK.

PE

129

Papular Urticaria

Hypersensitivity Reactions to Arthropod Bites

The bites of many arthropods can trigger hypersensitivity reactions in humans. This chapter discusses those hypersensitivity reactions to arthropod bites from species that do not live on humans. (Scabies and lice are discussed in Chs. 156 and 132, respectively.) By far the most common are mosquito bites, followed by bites by fleas, chiggers, and blackflies ("no-see-ems"). Many of these arthropods have pets or other animals as their primary host (e.g., *Cheyletiella*, animal scabies, some fleas). All these bites result in similar urticarial pruritic lesions called *papular urticaria.*

Initial Therapy

1. The most difficult step in therapy is identifying the offending arthropod: three factors are needed in this identification:
    a. Know the biting arthropods in your geographic region.
    b. Know the distribution pattern of bites (i.e., lower leg: fleas, chiggers; exposed areas of arms and face: biting flies, mosquitos).
    c. Take a careful history from the patient: Are there pets in the home? Have arthropods been seen or collected? Is there occupational/ recreational exposure? In difficult cases, this information is critically important, and aids in identifying unusual causes of papular urticaria (e.g., rat mite dermatitis).
2. Exclude human scabies and lice infestation by careful examination of the patient's body and clothing.
3. Management involves three basic steps:
    a. Treat the patient's hypersensitivity reaction:
        (i) Oral antihistamines (e.g., hydroxyzine 25–50 mg q.h.s. and 10–25 mg t.i.d. steadily for 1 week). The nightly dose is *not* given p.r.n., but rather is given *every* night, so the antihistamine is "on board" when a bite occurs in order to block the allergic cascade induced by the bite.
        (ii) Apply a high- to superpotency topical steroid b.i.d. to t.i.d. to each new papule until it resolves.
        (iii) Secondary infection is common; treat it with appropriate antibiotics (e.g., oral dicloxacillin 250 mg q.i.d. for 7 days).
    b. Make the patient less attractive to the biting arthropod:
        (i) Instruct the patient to apply an insect repellant containing diethyltoluamide (DEET) daily:
        (ii) Avon's "Skin So Soft" body lotion has been reported as a cosmetically acceptable insect repellent;
        (iii) When outdoors, cover as much exposed skin as possible.
    c. Instruct the patient to eliminate infestations of pets and/or the environment: A veterinarian and a professional exterminator may be helpful in this endeavor. The basic principles of flea control are discussed here, as this is one of the most common problems.
        (i) Treat all dogs and cats in the household. Cats especially may harbor fleas without visible signs. Flea collars and ultrasonic

devices are inadequate. Bathe the pet with a flea shampoo to kill the infesting fleas, then dip the animal in an effective agent (e.g., Paramite, Ectoral).

(ii) Spray or wash the bedding on which the pets sleep or lie for significant periods.

(iii) If the pet frequently lies in one area outdoors, treat this area with an effective insecticide (e.g., malathion, diazinon). It is probably not necessary to treat the entire yard, although this can be done and should be considered in situations of severe hypersensitivity.

(iv) Use flea bombs (foggers) in all the rooms of the house, especially carpeted areas. Most effective are those containing an agent that kills adult fleas (e.g., pyrethrin) plus an insect growth regulator to stop development of immature forms (e.g., fenoxycarb or methoprene). Additional spraying may be required under furniture and in crevices along the wall boards.

(v) Vacuum the entire house and all furniture to pick up eggs and adults. Dispose of the vacuum bags immediately after vacuuming

Subsequent Therapy

1. Most patients who fail to respond to the above measures are still being bitten. Additional effort to remove the cause of the papular urticaria should be undertaken. The patient should consult an exterminator and have pets examined by a veterinarian.

2. Rare patients will require a short course of systemic steroids for severe reactions.

3. More powerful antihistamines (e.g., doxepin 25–50 mg q.h.s.) may be quite helpful. They should be continued as suppressive therapy for as long as lesions persist.

4. For flea control, the pets and environment must be repeatedly treated, initially 1–2 weeks after the first treatment, and then as frequently as biweekly depending on the level of infestation and severity of reaction. Flea powders and sprays may be used on pets if dipping is not possible. Frequent vacuuming helps reduce the flea population.

Pitfalls

1. Misdiagnosis is the major pitfall. Patients with papular urticaria are frequently misdiagnosed as having human scabies. Frequent applications of lindane exacerbate the hypersensitivity reaction.

2. Delusions of parasitosis presents with *no* primary lesions, but a strong story of infestation (see Ch. 42, Delusions of Parasitosis).
3. Doxepin is a tricyclic antidepressant, and must be used with care in patients with cardiac disease or those who are suicidal risks.
4. Most pesticides are toxic. Repeated or incorrect use can produce toxicity. Follow directions carefully.
5. Do not rule out papular urticaria if only limited members of a family are affected. Because papular urticaria is a hypersensitivity reaction, only sensitized household members will have clinical lesions, even though all family members are bitten.

TB

130

Paronychia

Paronychia is inflammation of the lateral or proximal nail folds. Toenail paronychia is usually acute, associated with an ingrown nail, and may have a component of bacterial overgrowth (see Ch. 96, Ingrown Nail). Fingernail paronychia is either acute or chronic. Acute paronychia may be caused by bacteria (staphylococci or streptococci) or *C. albicans.* To distinguish, a Gram stain and a KOH preparation of any recovered purulent material should be performed. Chronic paronychia is associated with wet work (bartenders, housewives) and diabetes, and is due to *C. albicans.*

Initial Therapy

BACTERIAL PARONYCHIA

1. Surgically drain any fluctuant areas.
2. Oral dicloxacillin 250 mg q.i.d. for 10 days.

CANDIDAL PARONYCHIA (ACUTE OR CHRONIC)

1. Surgically drain fluctuant areas.
2. Lotrimin 1% solution t.i.d. Response is slow (weeks to months).
3. Keep hands out of water as much as possible. Stop all manicuring.

Alternative Therapy

BACTERIAL PARONYCHIA

Acute bacterial paronychia that is progressing associated with cellulitis, or accompanied by significant pain, fever, or an elevated WBC may be an indication for hospitalization and intravenous antibiotic therapy.

CANDIDAL PARONYCHIA

1. Thymol 2%–4% in chloroform or ethanol up to q.i.d.
2. If onycholysis is present, trim back the nail plate to the point of attachment.
3. For severe recalcitrant cases, oral ketaconazole 200–400 mg/day for several weeks.

Pitfalls

1. Tinea almost never causes paronychia. Think of something else.
2. Bacterial paronychia may quickly progress to a felon.
3. Combined bacterial and candidal infection may occur, requiring therapy for both.
4. Chronic paronychia frequently relapses, but is usually multifocal. If one area remains chronically inflamed a biopsy should be performed to rule out a malignancy.
5. Chronic paronychia, especially unassociated with significant water exposure, should prompt an evaluation for diabetes mellitus.
6. Oral ketaconazole may be associated with elevated LFTs.

TB

131

Parapsoriasis

Chronic Superficial Dermatitis • Digitate Dermatosis

This benign disorder is usually unaccompanied by symptoms and responds poorly to therapy. It should not be confused with forms of parapsoriasis that may herald development of cutaneous T-cell lymphoma (see Ch. 39). Because no form of therapy is clearly superior, therapeutic alternatives are listed and described.

Therapeutic Alternatives

1. No treatment. Because the disorder is benign and does not easily respond to safe therapies, it is reasonable to reassure and educate the patient while leaving the condition untreated.
2. Topical steroid therapy. Apply a medium-potency fluorinated steroid (e.g., triamcinolone 0.1% cream or ointment) with or without liquor carbonis detergens 10% b.i.d. If a favorable response does not occur in 3–4 weeks, elect another modality or discontinue treatment.
3. Ultraviolet light therapy. UVB phototherapy may be attempted 3×/week for 3–4 weeks, with or without a topical tar preparation applied 60 minutes prior to light exposure. The UVB dose must be individualized and gradually increased. If the patient responds, gradually reduce UVB therapy to the amount necessary to maintain remission. Discontinue therapy if no response is noted after 6 weeks.
4. Other alternatives. Multiple modalities have been tried, including antimalarials and photochemotherapy (PUVA). However, the use of even these relatively benign modalities is difficult to justify, as a satisfactory clinical response is unlikely.

Pitfalls

This disorder may be confused with other less-benign disorders that are also called parapsoriasis. For this reason, biopsy is recommended to confirm the diagnosis, and the patient should be seen yearly to ascertain that the process has not changed.

BW

132

Pediculosis (Lice)

Humans may be parasitized by three louse types: body lice, head lice, and pubic lice. Body lice live in the patient's clothing, not on the body. Head and pubic lice are found on the hair of the scalp and genital area, respectively. Pubic lice may also infest the eyelashes.

Initial Therapy

BODY LICE

1. All of the patient's infested clothing and bedding is disposed of if possible. The remaining bedding and clothes is washed in very hot water and the seams ironed. Clothes may be dusted with malathion 1% powder.
2. The patient bathes well with soap and water.
3. Lindane lotion can be used if nits are found on the body, but this is usually unnecessary.
4. Topical steroids and oral antihistamines are often required for days to weeks to control the pruritus.

HEAD LICE

1. Permethrin 1% rinse (NIX) is applied for 10 minutes after shampooing, then rinsed off.
2. For cosmetic reasons it is best to comb out nits with a fine-toothed comb, after applying a dilute (50%) vinegar solution to the scalp.
3. Examine and treat other infested contacts.

PUBIC LICE

1. Lindane shampoo is applied in the shower for 5 minutes, or lindane lotion is applied for 12 hours followed by a thorough washing. In hairy persons treat not only the genital area, but as far as infestation is found.

2. For eyelash pediculosis, petrolatum is applied 3–5×/day for 10 days. As many nits and lice are removed mechanically as possible.
3. Treat all infested contacts.
4. Examine the patient for other STDs, especially gonorrhea and syphilis.
5. Refer children with pubic lice for evaluation for sexual abuse.

Alternative Therapy

HEAD LICE

1. RID or A-200 pyrinate (synergized pyrethrins) are over-the-counter products that are very effective. They are applied for 10 minutes, then rinsed off. Treatment may be repeated in 1 week.
2. Lindane shampoo is applied for 10 minutes, then rinsed off.
3. Crotamiton 10% lotion is applied to scalp for 24 hours.
4. Malathione 0.5% lotion (Priderm) is left on for 12 hours, then washed off.

PUBIC LICE

1. RID is applied for 10 minutes, then washed off. A repeat treatment may be needed in 1 week.
2. For eyelash pediculosis: physostigmine ophthalmic ointment is applied several times daily for 3 days; or fluorescein eyedrops (20%) are applied to the lid margins once (may be repeated in 10 days); or yellow oxide of mercury 1% ophthalmic ointment or ammoniated mercury 3% ophthalmic ointment is applied b.i.d. for 1 week.

Subsequent Therapy

1. All patients infested with lice should be reexamined after 1 week. If active infection is still present repeat the initial therapy and suspect reinfection. Carefully examine contacts.
2. Sulfamethoxazole-trimethoprim is an effective oral pediculocide when ingested for at least 1 week. It should be used only in refractory cases owing to potential adverse reactions.

Pitfalls

1. Lindane is an irritant, and aggressive overuse can lead to dermatitis and pruritus. This is especially true in those with established dermatitis from pediculosis.
2. Lindane should not be used in pregnant women, if avoidable, and in children under 6 years of age.

3. Lindane resistance is usually a problem only with head lice. More effective alternatives are preferred as initial therapy.

TB

133

Pemphigus Foliaceus

Pemphigus Erythematosus

Pemphigus foliaceus is relatively benign, and is characterized by circulating and deposited autoantibodies. The therapeutic approach differs significantly from that for pemphigus vulgaris (Ch. 134), and therapy is adjusted on the basis of clinical response rather than immunopathologic data. The goal is to control blister formation, although an occasional blister should be tolerated, as chronic effects of therapy may be more dangerous than the disease. Pemphigus erythematosus may be treated like pemphigus foliaceus.

Initial Therapy

1. Treat with prednisone 60 mg/day.
2. If possible, apply a superpotent topical steroid cream s.i.d. to b.i.d. to each lesion.
3. Expect disease suppression within 2–3 weeks.

Subsequent Therapy

1. Continue administration of superpotent topical steroid.
2. Reduce the prednisone q.d. dose by 10 mg/week until 20 mg/day is reached. Then reduce by 5 mg q.o.d. until 20 mg q.o.d. is achieved. Then reduce by 2.5 mg/week.
3. Use the lowest prednisone dose needed for maintenance.

Alternative Therapy

1. Add azathioprine (Imuran) 100 mg/day to the regimen for patients who are not controlled with q.o.d. doses of prednisone.
2. Consider starting therapy with azathioprine 100 mg/day and prednisone 60 mg/day in patients with extensive disease.
3. Use only topical steroid therapy for patients with mild disease.
4. Intramuscular methotrexate 25–50 mg/week, oral cyclophosphamide 75–150 mg/day, and dapsone 100 mg/day have been used in combination with prednisone.

Pitfalls

1. Drugs such as penicillamine and captopril may cause pemphigus foliaceus. These should be discontinued. Most drug-induced cases can be treated with superpotent topical steroids.
2. Pemphigus foliaceus may rarely be associated with lupus erythematosus. This disorder is called *pemphigus erythematosus*, and is treated like pemphigus foliaceus.

BW

134

Pemphigus Vulgaris

Because overwhelming evidence suggests a cause and effect relationship between pemphigus autoantibody and the disease process, therapy is aimed at both resolution of cutaneous lesions and elimination of circulating antibody. The life-threatening nature of pemphigus mandates aggressive therapy.

Initial Therapy

1. Treat with prednisone 60–100 mg/day in combination with azathioprine (Imuran) 100 mg/day.
2. Demonstrate in vivo bound immunoreactants by direct immunofluorescence, and quantitate circulating pemphigus antibodies by indirect immu-

nofluorescence. Repeat indirect immunofluorescence every 4 weeks, and watch for a fall in antibody titer.
3. To reduce gastric-peptic ulceration caused by systemic steroids, encourage a bland diet and antacids between meals.
4. Follow patients closely and look for suppression of new blister formation.
5. Stop drugs known to induce pemphigus vulgaris, such as penicillamine, captopril and rifampin.

Subsequent Therapy

1. After pemphigus is under control (6–8 weeks):
   a. Monitor serum antibodies. When circulating pemphigus antibodies disappear from the serum, re-examine the skin for their presence by direct immunofluorescence.
   b. After pemphigus antibodies disappear from serum and skin, slowly taper prednisone by 2.5–5 mg/week.
   c. After prednisone has been discontinued, taper azathioprine over a 1–2-month period.
   d. After discontinuation of drugs, observe at 3–4-month intervals.
2. If pemphigus is not controlled after 6–8 weeks:
   a. Increase prednisone to 120–150 mg/day;
   b. Observe for another 6–8 weeks. When pemphigus is controlled, begin reducing medication as described above.

Alternative Therapy

1. Intramuscular methotrexate 25–50 mg/week, or oral cyclophosphamide 75–150 mg/day may be substituted for azathioprine.
2. Some clinicians use gold 25–50 mg/week (up to a total dose of 1,500 mg) as initial therapy, or in steroid- or immunosuppressive-resistant patients.
3. Removal of pemphigus antibodies by plasmapheresis is a promising therapy, which may be useful in combination with steroids or immunosuppressives. Three to six plasma exchanges over 2–3 weeks are appropriate. Plasmapheresis has been used in patients who do not adequately respond to steroids and immunosuppressives.
4. Dapsone 100 mg/day has been used in combination with prednisone and would be appropriate in patients who do not tolerate other proven agents.
5. Photopheresis has been used in difficult cases.

Pitfalls

1. Before beginning steroid-immunosuppressive therapy, examine patients for contraindications to such therapy.
2. In the presence of a history of tuberculosis, treat concomitantly with oral isoniazid 300 mg/day throughout steroid or immunosuppressive therapy.
3. Closely follow patients for clinical complications of immunosuppression and high-dose steroid therapy (see Appendices 5 and 7).
4. Topical therapy is generally not useful.

BW

135

Periarteritis Nodosa

Polyarteritis Nodosa

Periarteritis nodosa (PAN) can be a multisystem disease or a localized process limited to one or more extremities, with local skin, muscle, or nerve involvement (cutaneous PAN). Certain infections and drugs also can induce a PAN-like syndrome.

Initial Therapy

1. Initially, perform a skin biopsy of an early lesion, extending through the subcutaneous fat. Histologic examination should show a necrotizing vasculitis of muscular arterioles, and in early lesions there should be evidence of immune complex deposition on immunofluorescence.
2. Systemic corticosteroids are usually effective, but long-term, high-dose therapy is often required (e.g., prednisone, 60 mg/day in divided doses for 3–6 months). The dose then is tapered slowly over several months. *Note:* Too-rapid tapering can result in flares, leading to unnecessary prolongation of corticosteroid therapy.
3. Patients presenting initially with PAN or PAN-like lesions should be checked for antecedent or concurrent streptococcal or hepatitis infection.

4. Chronic drug reactions can present with PAN-like lesions. Hence, for new cases of PAN receiving potentially offending agents (e.g., iodides, thiazides, barbiturates) withdraw the drug(s) and substitute non-cross-reacting agents.

Ancillary Therapy

1. Nicotinic acid 100 mg t.i.d., taken immediately after meals, can be effective alone, and also can be used in conjunction with corticosteroids to reduce dosages of the latter. *Note:* Try nicotinic acid alone, prior to initiation of corticosteroid therapy, in cases of cutaneous PAN.
2. Chronic ulcerations, usually on the leg, can occur in PAN. Treat these lesions with soaks, topical antimicrobials, and vapor-permeable membranes.

Alternative Therapy

1. Dapsone 50 mg b.i.d. or sulfapyridine 500 mg q.i.d. may be effective in PAN, and should be used in patients who either are unresponsive to or cannot receive systemic corticosteroids. Again, therapy should be combined with niacin, as above.
2. Cyclophosphamide (Cytoxan) 2 mg/kg/day, alone or in combination with low-dose steroids, may be useful and help to reduce steroid dosages.
3. A combination of aspirin 300 mg b.i.d. and dipyridimole (Persantine) 25 mg q.i.d., increasing to 200–300 mg/day, has been reported to benefit the livedoid lesions in cutaneous PAN.
4. For nonhealing leg ulcers: hyperbaric oxygen may be helpful as a last resort, prior to amputation.
5. Although plasmaphoresis has not been shown to benefit PAN, it should be tried in patients refractory to the other forms of therapy described above.

Pitfalls

1. The hazards of too-rapid tapering of systemic corticosteroid therapy are detailed above.
2. The possibility of a reversible cause of PAN (e.g., from infection or drug reaction) should not be overlooked.
3. The pitfalls of systemic corticosteroids are described in Appendix 5.
4. The pitfalls of therapy with sulfones are described in Chapter 84.
5. The pitfalls of immunosuppressive therapy are described in Appendix 7.
6. Although nicotinic acid can produce uncomfortable flushing reactions, tolerance usually develops. The use of a divided-dose regimen, ingestion at

the end of meals, and low doses of aspirin all can alleviate flushing. *Note:* Nicotinic acid must be used with caution in patients with possible or known coronary artery disease.

PE

136

Perioral Dermatitis

This form of acne is almost always related to the use of moderate to potent topical steroids in the affected areas (see Ch. 154, Rosacea).

Initial Therapy

1. Stop the offending topical steroid. Warn the patient that the condition will worsen after a few days to a week.
2. Administer oral tetracycline 250 mg b.i.d. for 4–8 weeks, then taper off over 2–3 months.
3. Desonide 0.05% cream or hydrocortisone 1%–2.5% cream may be used for the first 2–3 weeks to blunt the exacerbation induced by stopping the stronger topical steroid.

Alternative Therapy

When tetracycline is contraindicated, as in pregnancy, try benzoyl peroxide 2.5% water-based gel q.o.h.s., plus topical erythromycin 2% solution b.i.d.

Subsequent Therapy

1. In patients failing to respond to low-dose tetracycline the dose may be increased, or minocycline 100 mg/day may be substituted.
2. A trial of discontinuation of fluoride-containing toothpastes is occasionally of benefit.
3. Advise the patient to use only noncomedogenic moisturizers and cosmetics.

Pitfalls

1. Yeast vaginitis is a common complication of oral tetracycline therapy.
2. Tetracycline and minocycline are contraindicated in pregnancy.

TB

137

Photosensitivity Dermatitis

Including Persistent Light Reaction • Actinic Reticuloid • Polymorphous Light Eruption • Photoallergic and Phototoxic Drug Reactions

These entities represent a group of diseases triggered by sunlight, often interacting with a systemic or topical photosensitizer. Unfortunately, a rash may persist long after the offending agent is withdrawn. Porphyrias, lupus erythematosus, and pellagrous dermatitis must be ruled out in all patients who develop a chronic course.

GENERAL THERAPY

Initial Therapy

1. In phototoxic or photoallergic drug reactions, the offending agent, which may include thiazide diuretics, sulfonamides (some food additives, such as cyclamates, are sulfonamides), quinidine, tetracyclines, captopril, etretinate, phenothiazines, NSAIDs, and sulfonylureas, must be identified.
2. Identification and removal of the offending allergen may be difficult because of the ubiquitous nature of some of these agents. Photopatch testing may be necessary in some cases (see below).
3. Encourage all patients with photosensitivity diseases to use an SPF 15 or higher sunscreen with ingredients that shield against both UVB and UVA

(e.g., Photoplex). In those patients sensitive to visible light, an opaque sunscreen (e.g., zine oxide or titanium dioxide) may be needed. Sunscreens should be applied q.a.m. and again after swimming, bathing, or extensive sweating.

4. Therapy of acute photoallergic dermatitis is the same as for acute contact dermatitis (see Ch. 34).
   a. Prescribe soaks (Burrow's solution, 1:10) to be applied t.i.d. for 15–20 minutes to areas of vesiculation, crusting, oozing, and/or secondary infection.
   b. Prescribe a high-potency steroid cream or gel such as fluocinolone to be applied to the rash t.i.d. after soaks.
   c. Give oral antihistamines such as hydroxyzine 10 mg q.i.d., increasing to 25 mg q.i.d., for cases accompanied by severe pruritus.

Additional Therapy

For severe disease, either a single intramuscular injection of triamcinolone acetonide (Kenalog) 40–80 mg or a 10–14-day tapering course of oral prednisone starting at 50–60 mg q.a.m. and decreasing by 5 mg/day.

PERSISTENT LIGHT REACTION AND ACTINIC RETICULOID

These patients are often severely disabled, and may require hospitalization. Actinic reticuloid is a persistent photosensitivity disorder in which patients respond abnormally to UVA, UVB, and sometimes to visible irradiation. The disorder is pruritic, and results in thick, lichenified photodistributed plaques with atypical histopathologic changes.

Initial Therapy

In addition to the measures described above (sunscreens, topical steroids, and occasional courses of systemic steroids), the following modalities may be tried in the order below:

1. Avoidance of UV irradiation, including fluorescent indoor lighting (using incandescent lamps only), is helpful but often impractical. For actinic reticuloid, a dark room may be required.

2. Beta-carotene (Solatene) 120–180 mg/day for adults, and 30–90 mg/day for children.
3. Photochemotherapy (PUVA) may be helpful, and should be tried prior to the next alternative. Start therapy very cautiously (0.1 to 0.25 J/cm^2) to limited parts of the body to avoid disease flares. The dosage can be slowly increased thereafter, maintenance therapy (1–2 ×/week) is needed even with clearing (see *Archives of Dermatologic Research* 269:87–91, 1980).
4. Azathioprine (Imuran) appears promising for some patients. Begin with 50 mg/day, increasing to 100–200 mg/day, as tolerated. If response is noted, continue azathioprine at the same dose until the process is controlled, then taper to the lowest level necessary to maintain clinical response. Check the CBC weekly or biweekly during azathioprine therapy (see Appendix 7).

POLYMORPHOUS LIGHT ERUPTION

Polymorphous light eruption tends to flare each spring, then spontaneously improve as tanning and/or "hardening" occur. For patients who do not develop hardening, all of the ancillary measures described below continue to apply.

Initial Therapy

1. The acute reaction is responsive to a high-potency topical steroid cream or gel (see Appendix 3). Reserve systemic steroid therapy for the most severe exacerbations.
2. PUVA is effective, but expensive, and is not always available. Instead, patients can be taught to self-melanize by ingesting trioxalen (Trisoralen) 20–30 mg/day 2 hours before gradually increasing periods of sun exposure (between 11 A.M. and 2 P.M.). Exposure starts with 10 minutes, increasing to 60 minutes in 10-minute increments. *Note:* Sunglasses are recommended to avoid possible long-term lens effects of UVA plus psoralens (formation of cataracts).

Alternative Therapy

For those patients not improving with melanization:

1. Give beta-carotene 3 mg/kg/day from March to October (depending on latitude; see below).
2. Hydroxychlorquine (Plaquenil) 200 mg b.i.d. may be tried in addition to beta-carotene from March to October.

Ancillary Measures

Even after identification and removal of the offending agent, patients must be informed that it can take weeks, months, or even years for photosensitivity to disappear. Advise patients to:

1. Avoid sun exposure between 9 A.M. and 4 P.M., particularly from March to October, and in semitropical or tropical latitudes. *Note:* Clouds are not a sunscreen.
2. Wear protective clothing (e.g., broad-brimmed hats, closely woven longsleeve shirts, and gloves).
3. Avoid prolonged exposure to fluorescent light sources.
4. Plan occupations and vacations based upon avoidance of the sun, if necessary.
5. Install plastic UV-opaque sheets on the inside of car windshields, and possibly house windows as well.
6. Avoid foods containing photosensitizers, such as celery, carrots, figs, and parsnips.
7. Use fragrance-free soaps and shampoos.

Subsequent Therapy

PHOTOPATCH TESTING

1. Photoallergens are found in cosmetics, herbal shampoos, household soaps, foods, sunscreens, and drugs. Photopatch testing performed by experts in this technique (usually in a tertiary care facility) may be necessary to identify the offending agent.
2. Light testing with artificial light sources to delineate the sensitivity spectrum may facilitate more precise use of sunscreens and more accurate patient education.

Pitfalls

1. Difficulty in identifying the responsible allergen.
2. Cross-reaction of certain nondrug food additives with drugs can cause confusing exacerbations or disease persistence.
3. Sunscreen agents themselves can be sensitizing. This may be extremely confusing if superimposed on the underlying disease. *P*-Aminobenzoic acids (PABAs) are much more commonly implicated, although benzophenones also cause allergic contact dermatitis.
4. Patients with persistent light reactions are often chronically depressed;

physicians must be aware of the social consequences of a disease that banishes patients to the night.

5. Check all patients with chronic photosensitivity for systemic lupus erythematosus and porphyria cutanea tarda.
6. Check patients with persistent light reaction or actinic reticuloid for the Sézary syndrome variant of cutaneous T-cell lymphoma.
7. PABAs may cross-react with thiazide diuretics, hence they should not be used in patients with photoallergic reactions from this drug.
8. PABAs also cross-react with benzocaine, procaine, P-phenylenediamine, and sulfanilamide. Hence, they should not be used in patients known to be allergic to one or more of these agents.
9. The pitfalls of chemotherapeutic agents, systemic steroids, and topical steroids are described in Appendices 3, 5, and 7.
10. The pitfalls of antimalarials are described in Chapter 48, Discoid Lupus Erythematosus.
11. The pitfalls of photochemotherapy are described in Chapter 147, Psoriasis.

PE

138

Pigmented Melanocytic Nevi

Including Dysplastic Melanocytic Nevi

Therapy for melanocytic nevi is determined by two factors: the risk for development of melanoma, and cosmetic appearance.

Initial Therapy

1. Refer patients with large congenital nevi (over 10 cm in diameter) to centers with experience in their management, as decisions must be made on a case-by-case basis.
2. Benign-appearing small congenital nevi (under 1.5 cm in diameter) can be observed until the patient reaches adulthood, when elective surgery can be considered. If changes occur during observation, consider excision.

3. Intermediate-sized congenital nevi should be evaluated initially by an expert, then followed.
4. Acquired nevi may be surgically excised or shave biopsied for cosmesis. Acquired nevi may occasionally develop a depigmented halo. Special evaluation is appropriate, especially when this occurs after age 20.
5. Make the diagnosis of dysplastic nevi based on both the clinical and histologic features of the lesions. Once the diagnosis is established:
    a. Categorize the patient by risk for development of melanoma.
        (i) *High risk:* Multiple dysplastic nevi and a family history or personal history of melanoma.
        (ii) *Intermediate risk:* Family history and/or personal history of multiple dysplastic nevi, but no melanoma.
        (iii) *Low risk:* Solitary dysplastic nevus.
    b. High-risk patients require skin examination by a skilled physician 2–4 X/year and regular photographs of their lesions; intermediate-risk patients should have skin examinations biannually, and low-risk patients once yearly.
    c. All patients should avoid sun and ultraviolet exposure, and use sunscreens.
    d. Because dysplastic nevi are familial, examine first-degree relatives, especially in the high- and intermediate-risk groups. Genetic counselling is appropriate in patients from melanoma-prone kindreds.
    e. Dysplastic nevi may recur after incomplete excision. In pathologically borderline lesions, re-excision with 0.5 cm (5 mm) of normal skin may be prudent.

Pitfalls

1. All biopsy material from pigmented skin lesions *must* be submitted to a competent laboratory for pathologic evaluation. Melanocytic nevi should never be electrosurgically destroyed without pathologic evaluation. Consultation with regional dermatopathology experts is required in borderline or atypical lesions. Pathologic misdiagnosis is a major potential liability, and it is the *clinician* who is responsible for ensuring that adequate and competent pathologic evaluation has been performed.
2. If melanoma is considered, an excisional biopsy of the suspicious lesion is highly recommended.
3. Compound nevi partially removed by shave biopsy may recur. These recurrent pigmented lesions may be clinically and pathologically quite atypical, and are easily misdiagnosed as melanoma.
4. Patients with a solitary dysplastic nevus (or no dysplastic nevi) may develop melanoma. Careful skin examination, especially of the high-risk

BANS areas (*b*ack, *a*rms, *n*eck, posterior *s*calp) and chest (and legs of women), should be performed once yearly in those at risk for melanoma by virtue of their skin type (fair), environmental exposure (excess sun exposure), nevus pattern (dysplastic nevi), and family history.

139

Pityriasis Rubra Pilaris

Pityriasis rubra pilaris (PRP) displays features of psoriasis and seborrheic dermatitis, but is more resistant to topical therapy. Spontaneous remissions occur within 2–4 years in most patients.

Initial Therapy

A 6–10-week course of oral systemic retinoids (isotretinoin, etretinate, or acitretin 2 mg/kg/day) will produce rapid, permanent clearing in about 50% of patients. A lesser percentage will improve partially, but not clear, requiring long-term maintenance therapy, and another group will not respond at all.

Subsequent Therapy

For thickened palms and soles: Either a 5% solution of flexible colloidion in ethyl acetate (keep sealed and refrigerated between uses) or flexible colloidion in zinc oxide paste applied q.a.m. can be used to coat painful fissures.

Alternative Therapy

1. Cytotoxic immunosuppressive agents, such as methotrexate 50 mg/week, in a single oral or intramuscular bolus initially followed by gradual tapering down to the lowest effective dose (usually around 10 mg/week).
2. Systemic and topical steroids help some patients.
3. Photochemotherapy (PUVA) or standard tar plus UVB phototherapy may help some patients.

4. In children with PRP, try topical retinoic acid (Retin-A) 0.05% cream, applied q.h.s. after bathing each morning, prior to administration of systemic retinoics, steroids, or chemotherapeutic agents.

Pitfalls

1. Second attacks or relapses of PRP may occur after complete clearing.
2. Occasionally, PRP may progress to a generalized, exfoliative erythroderma that can persist for years and be completely recalcitrant to all forms of therapy.
3. The thickened palmar/plantar hyperkeratosis of patients with PRP is difficult to treat, and can present occupational problems as well.
4. For pitfalls of systemic retinoid therapy, see Appendix 6.
5. For pitfalls of systemic steroids, see Appendix 5.
6. For pitfalls of cytotoxic agents, see Appendix 7.

PE

140

Porokeratosis

Initial Therapy

1. Topical 5-fluorouracil (5-FU) 5% cream applied q.d. or b.i.d. to lesions, until the epidermis desquamates and a crust forms, will often resolve superficial lesions. On thick-skinned areas, retinoic acid 0.1% cream, or salicylic acid 6% gel, may be added to enhance effect. Treatment usually requires at least 3–6 weeks.
2. Surgical excision or electrodesiccation may be used for small lesions. Carbon dioxide laser has also been reported to be as effective.
3. Counsel patients with lesions in sun-exposed areas to avoid the sun, and to use sunscreens of SPF 15 or greater.

Alternative Therapy

Although systemic retinoids may be effective the therapy is rarely indicated, as the disease is minimally symptomatic, and the doses required usually lead to retinoid toxicity (see Appendix 6 for effects of systemic retinoids).

Subsequent Therapy

1. Porokeratosis may be premalignant. Any papule, nodule, or ulcer developing in association with a lesion of porokeratosis must be biopsied.
2. Porokeratosis is an autosomally dominantly inherited genetic trait. Genetic counselling is appropriate.

Pitfalls

1. The diagnosis of porokeratosis should be confirmed by biopsy prior to initiating therapy.
2. Topical 5-FU therapy can cause severe skin inflammation. Patients must be carefully counselled and regularly followed during treatment.
3. Surgical therapy usually results in scarring.

TB

141

Porphyria Cutanea Tarda

Initial Therapy

1. Stop exacerbating drugs (estrogens, OCPs, iron) or chemicals (pesticides, herbicides).
2. Counsel the patient to stop *all* alcohol ingestion.
3. Inform the patient that sunlight is a cofactor, and have the patient *protect his skin from the sun* until therapy has lowered his porphyrin levels. Sunscreens are inadequate. Opaque physical blocks are required.
4. Obtain a baseline 24-hour urine quantitative porphyrins to guide therapy.
5. Evaluate for hepatocellular disease with a physical examination and LFTs. Acute hepatitis and hepatoma may precipitate porphyria cutanea tarda.
6. In the nonanemic patient, repeated venesection of 400–500 ml of blood every 2–4 weeks may be performed. Hospitalized patients may have more frequent phlebotomies.

Alternative Therapy

1. Low-dose chloroquine 125 mg 2×/week is quite effective. Check the LFTs, then give a test dose of chloroquine 125 mg, and recheck the LFTs before instituting therapy.
2. Porphyria cutanea tarda patients on dialysis may be treated with desferoxamine. This drug may increase the risk for opportunistic fungal infections.

Subsequent Therapy

1. Phlebotomy is continued until clinical improvement occurs, keeping the hemoglobin in the 10–11-g range. Urine porphyrins fall with phlebotomy and may continue to fall for months after phlebotomy is discontinued.
2. Chloroquine therapy is continued until urinary porphyrins are less than 300 mg/24 hrs. Monitor LFTs monthly.

Pitfalls

1. Do *not* give iron to correct the anemia induced by phlebotomy.
2. Higher doses of chloroquine may induce a severe hepatotoxic crisis, with fever, chills, vomiting, and elevated LFTs.
3. A clinically and histologically identical syndrome with normal porphyrins (pseudoporphyria) may be induced by certain phototoxic agents, notably tetracycline and naproxen. Urinary porphyrins are required to establish the correct diagnosis. Patients on dialysis may develop true porphyria or pseudoporphyria. Plasma and stool porphyrin levels are needed for diagnosis in this setting.
4. Nonopaque sunscreens are *not* protective, as the active spectrum is at 400–410 nm, the borderline of long UV and visible violet radiation (Soret band).

TB

142

Pretibial Myxedema

Although usually associated with hyperthyroidism, pretibial myxedema may appear long after the thyroid disease has been treated and the patient is euthyroid.

Initial Therapy

1. High-potency to superpotent topical steroids may considerably improve or eliminate lesions. Occlusion may enhance the efficacy and may be added if there is no initial response. Do not continue occlusion beyond 2 weeks.
2. Evaluate for and treat underlying thyroid disease.

Alternative Therapy

Intralesional triamcinolone acetonide 5 mg/cc will reduce plaques.

Subsequent Therapy

Lesions failing to respond to topical steroids usually respond to intralesional steroid therapy.

Pitfall

See Appendices 3 and 4 for complications of topical and intralesional steroids.

TB

143

Prurigo Nodularis

This severely pruritic disorder is often very difficult to manage, especially if there is an associated psychological disorder.

Initial Therapy

1. Prescribe high-potency to superpotent topical steroids to be applied b.i.d. to q.i.d. *with* occlusion.
2. If there are only a few lesions, intralesional triamcinolone acetonide 5–10 mg/cc to the mid-dermis of the lesion is often of great benefit.
3. Hydroxyzine or diphenhydramine 25–75 mg q.h.s. and as tolerated t.i.d.
4. During the *initial* visit an assessment of the patient's mental status is essential. Angry or depressed patients and those with obvious psychiatric disease often need a combined psychocutaneous approach for therapy to be effective.

Subsequent Therapy

1. If occlusion with superpotent steroids and/or intralesional therapy fails, consider covering the extremity with an occlusive dressing (e.g., an Unna boot) for 1–2 weeks. If the patient does not remove the dressing or manipulate the lesions beneath it with a coat hanger or other device, the lesions usually will improve.
2. If standard antihistamines are of no benefit, antianxiety agents (e.g., alprazolam [Xanex]) or tricyclics (e.g., doxepin [Adapin, Sinequan]) may help. Doses required may be above the standard doses prescribed for pruritus.
3. Thalidomide in doses of 100–400 mg/day is reported as beneficial, but is not readily available for this indication in the United States or Canada.

Pitfalls

1. Polymorphous light eruption, especially in Native Americans, may appear identical to prurigo nodularis on the extensor surfaces of the upper extremities. Hypertrophic lichen planus, lichen amyloidosis, and discoid lupus erythematosus also may be clinically similar.

2. Lesions similar to prurigo nodularis can occur in occasional patients with bullous pemphigoid.
3. See Appendices 3 and 4 for complications of topical and intralesional steroids.
4. Thalidomide is a potent teratogen and may cause neuropathy. It should only be used in otherwise unmanageable patients, by those skilled in its use, and never in women of child-bearing potential.

TB

144

Pruritus Ani

In the absence of a primary cutaneous disorder, pruritus ani is thought to be caused by irritation from rectal mucus and fecal material. Accordingly, the therapeutic goal is relief of symptoms and control of irritation.

Initial Therapy

1. Perianal and anal hygiene after defecation is critical. After defecation, the patient should clean by washing with a mild soap and water and dry by patting (not wiping) the perianal area with soft toilet paper. Use of pre-moistened pads (Tucks) may be substituted for washing.
2. The perianal area should be kept dry with applications of Zeasorb powder as needed.
3. Treat perianal area with iodochlorhydroxyquin 3% and hydrocortisone 1% cream (Vioform-Hydrocortisone) or hydrocortisone and pramoxine 1%–2.5% cream (Pramosone) after perianal cleansing and b.i.d.
4. Soft, loose-fitting, natural-fiber underclothing should be worn; men should wear loose trousers and cotton boxer undershorts.

Subsequent Therapy

The patient should expect symptomatic relief within 10–14 days and then:

1. Continue perianal hygiene.
2. Apply Zeasorb powder as needed.
3. Decrease applications of iodochlorhydroxyquin 3% and hydrocortisone 1% cream or hydrocortisone and pramoxine 1%–2.5% cream to as infrequently as needed to control symptoms.
4. Continue wearing soft, loose-fitting, natural-fiber undergarments and, when possible, loose clothing.

Alternative Therapy

1. For severe cases with accompanying dermatitis, applications of a fluorinated steroid in a cream base b.i.d. may be necessary. Treat for no longer than 7–10 days. Under no circumstances should patients use fluorinated steroids in the perianal region on a chronic basis.
2. Balneol or Neutrogena soap may be used as adjuncts to the perianal hygiene program.
3. Application of an imidazole cream b.i.d. may be useful as empiric treatment for symptoms owing to suspected candidiasis.
4. Dietary alterations may be useful.
   a. Avoidance of milk, pork, corn, nuts, coffee, tea, cola, chocolate, alcohol, citrus fruits, and spices has been advocated.
   b. If necessary, dietary habits should be modified to encourage "regular" stool habits in order to avoid the irritation of constipation or frequent loose stools.
5. Oral nystatin (Mycostatin) tablets (500,000 U t.i.d.) may alleviate symptoms in difficult cases in which pruritus caused by yeast is suspected.

Pitfalls

Failure to detect a primary disease responsible for pruritus is the principal pitfall. Pinworms, tinea, candidiasis, erythrasma, diabetes, hemorrhoids, and psoriasis must be sought prior to therapy or in difficult cases.

BW

145

Pruritus Vulvae

True pruritus vulvae is the persistence of itching in the absence of a primary dermatologic disorder. For this reason, the therapeutic goal is to relieve symptoms and/or skin changes that result from chronic scratching and rubbing.

Initial Therapy

1. In the absence of clinical evidence of inflammation, treatment is primarily symptomatic and focuses on the vaginal environment.
    a. The vaginal area is carefully washed with an unscented soap (Neutrogena is excellent) and *patted* dry with a soft towel.
    b. Zeasorb powder is applied p.r.n. to maintain a dry environment.
    c. Soft, loose-fitting, natural-fiber clothing is worn to avoid mechanical irritation.
    d. All possible contact sensitizers or topical agents should be eliminated. These may include douches, spermicides, perfumes, feminine hygiene agents, and topical anesthetics.
2. If clinical evidence of dermatitis is present, treat affected area with a potent fluorinated steroid in a cream base for no longer than 7–10 days.
3. Treat with hydroxyzine (Atarax) 25–50 mg t.i.d. to q.i.d.
4. Perform a pelvic examination to rule out vaginitis from *Candida*, *Trichomonas*, or bacteria. Also evaluate for pinworms if pruritus ani coexists.

Subsequent Therapy

1. Gentle vaginal washing, application of Zeasorb powder, and wearing of soft, loose-fitting, natural-fiber clothing is continued.
2. A topical lotion (e.g., Sarna lotion) which relieves itching is applied.
3. Hydrocortisone 1% cream or hydrocortisone-pramoxine 1% or 2.5% cream (Pramosone) may be applied on a regular or as-needed basis.

Alternative Therapy

1. Empiric treatment with oral ketoconazole 2% cream (Nizoral) applied b.i.d. for 10 to 14 days or 200 mg/day for 14 days is advocated by some.
2. A single intramuscular dose of triamcinalone acetate (Kenalog) 40–60 mg,

or a single course of oral prednisone 30–60 mg/day for 5–7 days, may be tried.
3. Administer a single intralesional injection with corticosteroids (Kenalog 3 mg/cc).
4. Topical hormonal therapy may be useful in cases of vulvar dystrophy and may be empirically attempted in the absence of objective findings.
   a. Testoserone 2% ointment in petrolatum applied t.i.d. for 6 weeks, then b.i.d. for 4 weeks.
   b. Progesterone ointment 200 mg in 2 oz. of hydrophilic ointment applied b.i.d. for 6 months.
5. Psychiatric disorders may be manifest as genital itching, and consultation should be obtained in selected patients who do not respond to topical, symptomatic treatment.

Pitfalls

1. Do not overlook primary dermatologic disorders that may cause symptoms (e.g., moniliasis, trichomoniasis, psoriasis, atopic dermatitis, seborrhea). These should be sought initially, and in cases that fail to respond to symptomatic treatment.
2. Chronic potent fluorinated steroid use must be avoided.

BW

146

Pseudofolliculitis Barbae

Razor Bumps

Pseudofolliculitis barbae (PFB) or razor bumps is a condition commonly affecting black men (and women). It is caused by shaving, and it resolves when shaving is stopped. There are several basic factors that make management less than ideal: First, no method of shaving works for all patients. Second, with time many patients learn the best technique for them, but often only after several unsuccessful, painful attempts. Finally, many PFB patients cannot be continuously "clean shaven," which may interfere with certain forms of employment. Severity of disease dictates therapeutic options.

Initial Therapy

1. For persons with moderate to severe PFB, no shaving is recommended. They are best served by always having a beard.
2. Patient education is a cornerstone of management and must be detailed, honest, and repeated on subsequent visits. Control, not cure, must be emphasized.
3. Daily lifting out of any ingrowing hairs with a needle, beard pick, or pointed toothpick is required. Brisk washing of the affected area with a Buf-Puf or face cloth may also dislodge early ingrowing hairs. *Do not pluck out hairs;* simply lift out the ingrowing end.
4. Topical agents like benzoyl peroxide (to dry up pustules), topical retinoic acid, or mild salicylic acid preparations may be of some additional benefit and may be added to the shaving regimen, described below.
5. Hydrocortisone 1% cream should be applied after shaving and up to b.i.d., no matter what shaving techique is used. It reduces beard irritation.
6. Persons with active pustulation or moderate to severe involvement, if they want to attempt shaving in the future, must first grow a beard for 2–12 weeks to allow the bumps already present to resolve. During this period aggressive dislodgement of ingrowing hairs is performed.
7. There are three basic forms of shaving available to the PFB patient: razors, depilatories, and clippers. Each method will be discussed in detail below. PFB patients must take time when shaving and follow instructions carefully.
    a. Razor shaving: One of three types of blade razors may be used: single-blade disposable, an adjustable razor set at the lowest setting (least close shave), or a foil-guarded system (PFB shaving system). All are effective, but the latter is probably the best. Razor shaving is usually effective in those with mild to moderate PFB. Electric razors are usually no better than blade razors.
   Detailed instructions on the correct techniques are essential:
    (i) Dislodge all ingrown hairs.
    (ii) Soak the beard with a shave cream for several minutes.
    (iii) Shave with the grain using even, smooth strokes. Do not press down with the razor.
    (iv) Do not stretch the skin when shaving.
    (v) Shave each area only once. Do not go back over areas to shave missed hairs.
    (vi) Shave often enough to keep the beard hair an optimal length: long

enough to be out of the follicle, but short enough to not be ingrowing. This varies from daily to every third day, depending on the rate of the beard growth of the patient.

b. Depilatory shaving: Two forms of depilatories are available: barium sulfide and calcium thiogylcolate. Depilatory shaving takes time, is smelly, and is *irritating*. Due to their inherent irritancy, depilatories can rarely be used more often than twice weekly. Repeated applications enhance irritancy. It is generally more effective than razor shaving in those with moderate to severe PFB.

Detailed instructions on the correct technique are essential:

   (i) Mix the powder with cool water and apply a thin coat to one-fourth to one-half of the beard area. Applying to the whole beard at one time may allow paste to remain on the skin too long before removal.

   (ii) Remove as soon as the beard hairs are dissolved, usually 2–3 minutes.

   (iii) Scrape off the paste with a moist spatula or tongue blade using short rapid strokes in the direction of beard growth.

   (iv) Wash the area *thoroughly* with cool water and soap to remove all residual paste. Residual depilatory will cause irritation.

   (v) Repeat steps (i)–(iv) on the remaining beard areas.

   (vi) Apply hydrocortisone 1% cream after shaving and b.i.d.

c. Clipper shaving: Most PFB patients will be able to trim their beard with a triple "0" (zero) barber clippers with good results. The result is approximately a 1/16-inch stubble ("5 o'clock shadow"). Certain patients with mild to moderate PFB may be able to shave closer, *after clipping*, with a rotary triple-headed razor. A preshave is recommended when using clippers or rotary shavers.

Pitfalls

1. PFB may be misdiagnosed as acne vulgaris, pyoderma, or razor "allergy." If there is any doubt refer the patient for evaluation.

2. Do not be disappointed by therapeutic failure. Work with the patient (and his employer if necessary), and individualize his shaving technique.

3. Postinflammatory hyperpigmentation may occur from the PFB, or from irritating topicals (i.e., depilatories, benzoyl peroxide, or retinoic acid).

TB

147

Psoriasis

Reiter's Syndrome

THERAPEUTIC MODALITIES

Many efficacious therapeutic modalities are available for treatment of the various clinical forms of psoriasis; each is useful and may be the appropriate initial therapy in a given situation. The format of this chapter is therefore organized differently from most of the other chapters. First, each therapy is described. Next, appropriate therapies are suggested for each clinical form of psoriasis. The following accepted therapies are appropriate in a variety of situations. Treatment of skin lesions in Reiter's syndrome is identical to psoriasis therapy.

Topical Therapy

Numerous topical agents are available. Topical therapy alone offers excellent control for many milder forms of psoriasis.

1. Bland emollients. Liberal use of emollients to coat the epidermis (most effective after adequate hydration) is a cornerstone of psoriasis therapy. Bathe or soak local lesions in warm water for 10–20 minutes, pat dry, and apply an emollient. Effective emollients include Eucerin, petrolatum, aquaphor and mineral oil. Emollients may be applied as often as necessary (b.i.d. use is usually acceptable to patients).
2. Keratolytics. These agents remove scale most effectively when used after adequate hydration.
   a. Salicylic acid 2%–6% in petrolatum is applied b.i.d. and is allowed to remain on the lesions.
   b. Keralyt, a salicylic acid 6% and propylene glycol 60% gel, is particularly useful for hyperkeratotic lesions of palms and soles. Soak the skin in water, apply gel, then occlude (overnight if possible) with plastic wrap, a bag, or a glove.

    c. Propylene glycol 40%–60% solution removes thick scale, but must be used with occlusion (see Occlusive Therapy, below, for a description).

    d. Urea 20%–40% in petrolatum may also be used with occlusion.

    e. Baker's P&S, a compound of phenol less than 1% and saline 20% in liquid petrolatum, is particularly useful for removing scalp scale. Shampoo before bedtime, then gently rub P&S directly into the wet scalp and cover scalp with a plastic shower cap. Sleep with the shower cap on. The next morning use a shampoo containing keratolytic agents and tar. Nightly therapy may be required for 10–14 days to remove scale; use as needed thereafter.

3. Topical steroids. These are probably the most commonly used agents for treatment of localized psoriatic lesions. Apply superpotent fluorinated steroids in an ointment base (clobetasol propionate 0.05% [Temovate] or betamethasone dipropionate 0.05% [Diprolene] q.d. or b.i.d.) to individual lesions. Occlusion enhances local penetration and efficacy. Expect resolution of lesions by 4 weeks. Use of superfluorinated steroids should be time-limited to prevent atrophy of treated skin. If localized lesions do not resolve completely, choose another therapeutic approach. These agents should not, in general, be used for therapy of generalized psoriasis.

4. Tar preparations. A great variety of tar-containing agents are available. The following is a partial listing:

    a. Crude coal tar is prepared in 1%–5% concentrations in petrolatum, aquaphor, or zinc oxide paste. Salicylic acid 2%–5% may be added to provide keratolytic action. Because these agents are quite messy, they are best used in a hospital or psoriasis daycare outpatient setting as a component of the Goekerman regimen (see below).

    b. Liquor carbonis detergens (LCD), an alcohol extract of tar, is directly applied to individual lesions or to the entire integument as a 10% concentration in hydrophilic creams and lotions (e.g., aquaphor, Lubriderm). When used as a primary therapeutic agent, apply 10% LCD b.i.d. When used in combination with UVB light therapy, apply 30–60 minutes prior to light exposure (see Phototherapy, below).

    c. Cosmetically acceptable tar preparations in creams or gels (e.g., Fototar, Estar, Psoragel) q.d. or b.i.d. are suitable for outpatient use either alone or in combination with UVB light therapy (see Phototherapy, below). They are not messy, and wash off easily.

    d. Tar-containing shampoos are useful for treatment of scalp psoriasis. Use these shampoos up to 20 minutes s.i.d. or p.r.n. to treat the scalp.

5. Anthralin is appropriate for both in- and outpatient management in various concentrations and formulations, including 0.1%, 0.25%, 0.5%, and

1.0% in cream (Drithrocreme) or ointment (Lasan, Anthroderm), with and without salicylic acid; paste may be compounded by pharmacies in 0.1%–5.0% concentrations. These agents may cause irritation and staining of treated skin.

    a. To treat individual psoriatic plaques, apply anthralin 0.1% paste to lesions. Since anthralins cause irritation and edema, ring each lesion with petrolatum or zinc oxide paste to prevent irritation of surrounding normal skin. Dust the treated plaques with talc and cover the area with tube gauze bandages for 4 hours. Remove anthralin with mineral oil containing 5% sodium lauryl sulfate. In the absence of irritation, increase anthralin concentration every 3–4 days to a maximum of 5% or until the lesion clears. Advise patients that lesions will stain purple, and normal skin and clothing will stain brown.

    b. Short-contact anthralin therapy uses high-concentration anthralin cream or ointment for short periods to decrease time to clearing and minimize irritation.

        (i) Start with anthralin 0.25% concentration. Use a disposable plastic glove to apply anthralin cream or ointment to lesions. Allow anthralin to remain on for 15 minutes. Shower, washing lesions with soap and water.

       (ii) If no irritation is noted after 1 week, increase anthralin concentration to 1%.

      (iii) Next, increase contact time by 15-minute increments each week to 60 minutes maximum. Continue therapy until lesions clear.

Occlusive Therapy

Local or whole-body occlusion enhances hydration of the epidermis and promotes cutaneous penetration of topically applied drugs (e.g., topical corticosteroids and keratolytics).

1. Whole-body occlusion. Apply topical medication (steroid and/or keratolytic agent) and clothe the patient in a plastic exercise or "sauna" suit (these may be obtained in sporting goods stores and some pharmacies). Occlude hands with plastic gloves and feet with plastic bags, and close with tape. Maintain occlusion overnight or for a minimum of 4–6 hours if tolerated (some patients cannot tolerate the discomfort caused by heat and damp). Some therapists ask that patients wear moist pajamas and cotton gloves under the plastic suit; although clearly efficacious, many patients do not tolerate this maneuver.

2. Localized occlusion. Occlude the hands with plastic gloves, the feet with

plastic bags, and larger areas such as forearm, lower leg, or scalp with plastic wrap; gently but firmly tape the edges closed to seal the plastic cover. Occlude overnight or for a minimum of 4–6 hours.

Intralesional Therapy

Intralesional corticosteroids are useful in the therapy of localized, persistent psoriatic plaques. Up to a total of 20 mg of an insoluble corticosteroid (e.g., triamcinalone acetonide (Kenalog) 2.5–10.0 mg/cc) may be injected at one visit without significant systemic effect. Give total upper limit (i.e., 20–40 mg) over a 2-month period.

1. Using a 30-gauge needle, inject 0.2–0.3 cc of Kenalog 2.5–10.0 mg/cc directly into multiple, ordered sites within several lesions, including centers and peripheries.
2. Sites may be reinjected after 4–6 weeks.
3. For a discussion of potential pitfalls, see Appendix 4.

Phototherapy

UVB light therapy should be administered by specialists in special phototherapy units or by individual practitioners skilled in this modality. The principles of UVB therapy are outlined. Two forms of ultraviolet light therapy are in general use: erythemogenic and suberythemogenic. Daily use of emollients is essential to the phototherapy regimen.

1. Erythemogenic UVB therapy. The lowest dose of light producing a barely perceptible erythema 24 hours after exposure is the minimal erythema dose (MED) of UVB light. The UVB MED differs in each patient, and should be determined before UVB therapy by titrating incremental UVB light exposure through a template with a series of small openings. Start UVB therapy just below the MED, increasing the dosage gradually until minimal erythema is maintained for 12–24 hours after each treatment. Outpatients should be treated 3×/week, and inpatients should be treated q.d. or b.i.d.; 20–30 treatments will be required to clear ordinary cases. In outpatient settings, apply an emollient or cosmetically acceptable tar preparation (e.g., Fototar, Estar, Psoragel) 30–60 minutes before therapy.
2. Suberythemogenic therapy uses the lowest dose of UVB commensurate with clinical improvement, thus limiting total UVB exposure and avoiding light-induced burns. It may be safely administered by a trained technician.

Emollients or tar preparations may also be used with this technique. The initial UVB dose should be 50% of the MED; subsequent doses are determined by assessment of clinical response. If lesions improve, do not increase the UVB dose. With lack of improvement or slowing of progress, gradually increase the UVB dose.

Photochemotherapy (PUVA)

Topical or oral administration of 8-methoxypsoralen (psoralen) and UVA radiation is the most widely accepted form of photochemotherapy (PUVA = psoralen + ultraviolet A). This therapy is efficacious, requiring 20–25 treatments to achieve clearing; patients may then require infrequent regular treatments to maintain clinical remissions. Shield the patient's eyes during treatment to minimize ocular side effects, and cover uninvolved skin. Instruct the patient to wear protective glasses for 12 hours following psoralen ingestion.

1. PUVA—systemic psoralen: Give psoralen 0.6 mg/kg 2 hours before UVA exposure. Begin UVA light exposure with 0.5–4.5 J/cm^2, depending on the patient's degree of melanization (skin type). Treat at 2–3-day intervals until clear.
2. PUVA—topical psoralen: Soak the patient for 15 minutes in a dilute solution (5 capsules (50 mg) oxsoralen ultra in a bathtub of water) of psoralen in bathwater for 30 minutes before UVA phototherapy; this is said to decrease the required therapeutic dose of UVA, but it requires a large tub. Topical UVA may also be used for treatment of localized areas such as the hands or feet. Soak hands or feet in psoralen (0.1% in 30% alcohol) or apply psoralen (0.1% in aquaphor) with a cotton-tipped applicator for 30 minutes before UVA exposure.

PITFALLS

1. Early side effects include nausea following psoralen administration, phototoxic erythema, pruritus, variable pigmentation, and occasional worsening of psoriasis.
2. Late side effects include skin carcinogenesis (rare), enhanced photoaging, pigmentary changes, and ocular damage. To minimize these effects, shield the patient's eyes and uninvolved skin during therapy, and warn the patient to wear protective glasses for 12 hours following psoralen ingestion.

Systemic Therapy

Many systemic agents are or have been used to treat psoriasis. Methotrexate, etretinate, and possibly hydroxyurea are accepted forms of therapy.

METHOTREXATE
Methotrexate is an effective agent with well-studied efficacy and toxicity. Its use is reasonably standardized.

1. Indications include psoriatic erythroderma; acute pustular psoriasis; localized pustular psoriasis; psoriatic arthritis; extensive psoriasis unresponsive to other, less toxic therapies; psoriasis that interferes with quality of life; and psychologically disabling psoriasis.
2. Contraindications include decreased renal function, significantly abnormal liver function, pregnancy or anticipated pregnancy, recent or active hepatitis, cirrhosis, excessive alcohol consumption, severe leukopenia, thrombocytopenia, anemia, active peptic ulcer, active severe infectious diseases, and an unreliable patient. HIV infection is a relative contraindication.
3. Pretherapy evaluation should include history and physical examination, CBC and platelet count, urinalysis, serum creatinine, BUN, LFTs, chest x-ray, and liver biopsy. Some clinicians perform liver biopsy after 4–6 weeks of methotrexate therapy; however, development of chronic liver toxicity would not yet be present after 4–6 weeks of methotrexate therapy, and nonresponders should be spared the potential morbidity of liver biopsy.
4. Therapeutic regimens: The goal of therapy is to achieve control, rather than complete clearing, at the lowest possible dose of drug.
   a. Test dose: To eliminate hematologic idiosyncratic reactions, give oral or intramuscular methotrexate 2.5 mg and check the CBC after 5–7 days; do not proceed if the WBC is depressed below normal.
   b. Divided oral dose: Administer three doses of methotrexate 2.5–5.0 mg q.12h. each week. Increase the dosage monthly as necessary to control the disease.
   c. Single dose: Weekly single doses of methotrexate 7.5–25 mg orally, or 7.5–50 mg intramuscularly, are appropriate. The dose should be increased on a biweekly basis in 2.5–5.0-mg increments as necessary until the disease is controlled.
5. Pitfalls of methotrexate therapy include the following:
   a. Blood counts should be monitored weekly during dosage escalation

and at monthly intervals when the dose is stabilized. Always obtain blood counts 1 week after drug administration.

b. LFTs should be obtained at 4-month intervals.

c. Because liver damage may occur in the absence of abnormal LFTs, liver biopsy should be obtained prior to therapy and after each 1.5 g of methotrexate administered.

ETRETINATE AND ACITRETIN

The retinoids etretinate and acitretin (Psoritane) are useful agents in the therapy of a variety of forms of psoriasis.

1. Etretinate and acitretin are indicated in pustular and erythrodermic psoriasis, and are useful adjunctive therapies in many but not all patients with plaque psoriasis.
2. Etretinate and acitretin should not be used in women of child-bearing potential or in patients with lipid abnormalities or active hepatitis.
3. Begin therapy at a dose of 0.5 mg/kg/day and increase to a maximum of 1.0 mg/kg/day. The therapeutic dose may be changed at one to three week intervals depending on the clinical situation and side effects encountered.
4. Pitfalls: Common reversible side effects include cheilitis, facial dermatitis, conjunctivitis, xerosis, dry mouth, scaling, and hair loss. Systemic problems include arthralgia, hyperlipidemia, transaminase elevation, and teratogenicity. See Appendix 6.

HYDROXYUREA

Hydroxyurea is used by some in combination with other therapies, but is infrequently used as a primary agent. Give 1000–1500 mg/day, and monitor the CBC weekly for suppression of the WBC and development of macrocytosis.

CYCLOSPORIN A

Cyclosporin A may be used to treat a variety of severe forms of psoriasis. The clinical response is often dramatic; however, this agent has significant associated toxicity.

1. Cyclosporin A is indicated in generalized plaque psoriasis, erythrodermic psoriasis, and psoriasis of the palms and soles.
2. Begin therapy at a dose of 10 mg/kg/day and continue treatment until the patient clears or is stably improved (1 to 3 weeks). Reduce dose to 3–5 mg/kg/day and maintain the patient on the lowest possible dose that maintains clinical benefit.

3. Cyclosporin A causes dose-related renal insufficiency, and renal function must be carefully evaluated before and during therapy. Determine BUN, serum creatinine, creatinine clearance, 24-hour urine protein, and urinalysis as well as cyclosporin A level before therapy. At weekly intervals until the lowest drug dose is attained, determine BUN, serum creatinine, cyclosporin level and urinalysis. Cyclosporin level must be obtained 12 hours after the drug is ingested. Follow these parameters and creatinine clearance on a regular but less frequent basis during maintenance therapy. A 30% rise in serum creatinine suggests renal toxicity.
4. If renal toxicity is detected, reduce or discontinue cyclosporin A. Consultation with a physician familiar with the use of this agent is advised.
5. Other potential problems include hyperuricemia and lymphomas. Cyclosporin A is contraindicated in women of child-bearing potential except under unusual circumstances.

Therapeutic Regimens

GOEKERMAN REGIMEN

This regimen has been frequently modified, and varies from practitioner to practitioner. Its basic tenets include repeated application of crude coal tar preparations accompanied by aggressive UVB therapy. This regimen is best suited to hospital and psoriasis day-care settings owing to the use of messy tars. The method described below is that used in the University of California, San Francisco, Psoriasis Treatment Center.

1. First expose the patient to whole-body UVB using the erythemogenic method.
2. Apply crude coal tar beginning with 2% ointment, sparing intertriginous areas; the patient should wear a soft cotton gown. Allow the tar preparation to remain on for 6–8 hours.
3. Increase the crude coal tar concentration to 5%, then 10%, and finally to 20% at 3–5-day intervals as tolerated; add either salicylic acid or lactic acid 2%–10% to the mixture if the lesions are hyperkeratotic.
4. Shower off the tar with soap and water, and then give the patient another whole-body exposure UVB treatment.
5. If tolerated, increase UVB exposure time daily, or with each treatment. When 4 minutes of whole-body exposure UVB can be tolerated, add quartz light therapy for localized recalcitrant areas s.i.d. or b.i.d.
6. For recalcitrant lesions apply anthralin 1%–3% cream or paste, with or without 3% salicylic acid, for 1 hour/day.
7. Apply LCD 20% in aquaphor to the entire skin at bedtime.

8. Using this regimen, most patients clear after 3–4 weeks. Clinical remission lasts months to years in many patients if regular out-patient UVB treatment is maintained in conjunction with LCD 20% in aquaphor applied at bedtime.

INGRAM REGIMEN

This regimen combines topical use of anthralin with UVB therapy, and is frequently used in England, where it originated. It is most suited to a day-care or inpatient setting.

1. Bathe the patient in a coal tar solution for 15 minutes, followed (after determining the MED) by whole-body suberythemogenic UVB light exposure.
2. Apply an initial dose of anthralin 0.1% paste with a spatula to all psoriatic plaques. Powder the paste with talc, and cover the entire body with a tubular netting suit. Remove the paste with mineral oil or soft paraffin after 6–24 hours.
3. Increase the UVB dose and anthralin concentration every 2–3 days.
4. Following resolution of psoriasis, maintain remission using regular UVB treatments.

TREATMENT OF PSORIASIS

Psoriasis presents in many different clinical forms. Any of the multiple therapeutic modalities may be effective in some patients but not in others. In addition, in most cases there is no commonly preferred form of therapy. Rather, the clinician is faced with many efficacious therapeutic options that must be tailored to the patient's clinical, social, and personal situation. Appropriate therapy for a given case may be attempted in the patient's home, in a psoriasis day-care center, or in the hospital. For this reason, useful therapeutic options are grouped as alternatives for each form of psoriasis. The reader is referred back to detailed descriptions of each modality above.

Therapy of Plaque Psoriasis

Plaque psoriasis is the most common form of psoriasis, presenting as either *localized* or *more generalized* disease. Therapeutic options are listed according to extent of psoriatic plaques. The therapy chosen must reflect the patient's expectation and ability to comply; do not embark on a complex program that the patient is unlikely to follow!

LOCALIZED PLAQUE PSORIASIS

1. Initiate a regimen of hydration and liberal use of emollients, and apply a super- or high-potency fluorinated topical corticosteroid in an ointment base (see Appendix 1) to each lesion on a q.d. or b.i.d. basis. The topical steroid may be combined with LCD and salicylic acid (LCD 10%/salicylic acid 3%/fluocinonide (Lidex) 0.05% ointment) for more rapid results. Expect resolution in 3–4 weeks, and maintain remission with daily hydration and emollients.
2. Recalcitrant, local lesions may be treated with intralesional corticosteroids. Lesions on the elbows and knees may benefit from this approach. Intralesional injection is particularly useful in patients who do not wish to undertake regular home, topical therapy.
3. As an alternative to intralesional steroids, apply a semipermeable occlusive dressing (e.g., Restore or Duoderm) to the lesion, leaving it on for 1 week; repeat the application until the lesion clears (6–8 weeks). Superpotent topical steroids may be applied prior to application of the dressing.
4. Anthralin is suitable for treatment of thick, recalcitrant plaques.
5. UVB light therapy may be given to localized lesions using a light box by shielding uninvolved skin, or by use of a quartz lamp.
6. Topical PUVA, applying psoralen only to involved skin, is efficacious.

PITFALLS

These are outlined above in the detailed description of each therapy and in Appendices 3, 4, and 5. Do not chronically treat with fluorinated steroids, even for localized lesions. If topical steroid therapy does not completely clear lesions, try another approach or refer the patient to a dermatologist skilled in the treatment of psoriasis.

GENERALIZED PLAQUE PSORIASIS

1. Goekerman regimen: Although safe and highly effective, the patient must commit 3–4 weeks to this program and so will usually be unable to work. This therapy can be given in an outpatient day-care setting and does not require overnight hospitalization; incapacitated patients, however, may require inpatient care.
2. Phototherapy with UVB, combined with use of a simple emollient, is safe

and effective. Patient inconvenience is minimal, and response is often gratifying but slow. Some patients benefit from a home UVB light source, which may be built or purchased.

3. Photochemotherapy (PUVA) is an effective therapy (with associated risks—see above) often used in patients who cannot realistically be treated with the Goekerman regimen, who fail UVB alone, or who do not wish a therapeutic trial of outpatient UVB.

4. Methotrexate is an excellent agent for otherwise healthy patients with significant disease who are unable to comply with the Goekerman regimen, UVB, and PUVA because of lifestyle.

5. Etretinate, although more useful in other forms of psoriasis, may benefit patients with plaque psoriasis who fail the standard therapies above. This drug, however, is stored in tissues for months to years, *is clearly teratogenic,* and should not be used by women of child-bearing potential (see Appendix 7).

6. Combination therapies may be appropriate for patients with severe plaque psoriasis. They include:
   a. Goekerman regimen and methotrexate.
   b. Goekerman regimen and hydroxyurea.
   c. UVB and methotrexate.
   d. All forms of phototherapy, UVB, Goekerman, and PUVA may be enhanced by addition of low-dose etretinate. Begin patients on etretinate 20 mg q.d. (to avoid etretinate cutaneous side effects) and increase the dose by 10–20 mg at 1-week intervals until mild secondary effects are noted. Continue etretinate at this dose throughout phototherapy. When the patient is clear, discontinue etretinate and maintain remission with outpatient UVB phototherapy.

7. Cyclosporin A is appropriate in patients with recalcitrant psoriasis.

Therapy of Scalp Psoriasis

MILD DIFFUSE SCALP PSORIASIS

1. Shampoo for 5–20 minutes with a shampoo containing tar and salicylic acid on a regular p.r.n. basis. A daily shampoo may be required initially, but the process may be controlled with less frequent but regular use.

2. Apply a medium- or high-potency topical steroid solution nightly on a regular basis; initial management may require nightly application. Triamcinolone acetonide 0.1% solution or lotion is usually satisfactory. However, stronger preparations such as Lidex solution or Diprosone lotion may be required. When the scalp clears, attempt control with shampoo alone or the lowest-strength steroid solution that will maintain remission.

LOCALIZED PLAQUES

1. Treat with the same regimen used for mild, diffuse disease.
2. If shampoo and topical steroids are not adequate, the following alternatives are reasonable:
   a. Apply Baker's P&S solution to the scalp nightly and cover the scalp with a plastic shower cap.
   b. Apply a salicylic acid and coal tar solution (T-Derm) to the scalp, and cover overnight with a shower cap.
   c. Inject lesions with Kenalog (up to 5 mg/cc). Do not use more than 1 cc per visit, and do not repeat more frequently than at 6-week intervals.

EXTENSIVE SEVERE SCALP PSORIASIS

Therapy may usually be given at home; however, use of messy topical preparations in difficult cases may require a day-care setting.

1. Apply a potent keratolytic (e.g., Baker's P & S solution) or a tar-keratolytic preparation (T-Derm) to scalp at night, and cover overnight with a shower cap.
2. In the morning, wet the scalp thoroughly in the shower, vigorously rub a tar shampoo into the hair, and cover with a warm moist towel. After 15–20 minutes, rinse out the shampoo in the shower.
3. After the thick scale is removed (3–7 days), apply a high-potency steroid solution (e.g., Lidex solution or Diprosone lotion) to lesions after shampooing.
4. In a day-care or hospital setting, other tar preparations may be used. Crude coal tar 5% with salicylic acid 5% or 10% ointment may be applied to the scalp prior to wrapping with a warm, moist towel. Alternatives include LCD 10% in Nutraderm Lotion or Oil of Cade.
5. For long-term management, use tar shampoos and high-potency steroids on a regular, as needed basis.

Therapy of Guttate Psoriasis

This type of psoriasis may follow streptococcal upper respiratory tract infection and is often self-limited, usually lasting 6–8 weeks; obtain a throat culture and treat if strep is found. Therapeutic alternatives include:

1. Therapy with bland emollients.
2. UVB therapy.

3. Goekerman treatment in a day treatment setting for the rare, recalcitrant case.

Therapy of Erythrodermic (Exfoliative) Psoriasis

INITIAL THERAPY

1. Hospitalize the patient in a comfortably warm environment (to limit loss of body heat) and carefully monitor for potential cardiovascular, thermoregulatory, fluid, and electrolyte problems.
2. Treat with aggressive emollient therapy. Expect improvement within 3–7 days.
    a. Soak in warm water containing Aveeno for 15–20 minutes b.i.d. to q.i.d.
    b. After soaking apply Eucerin cream.

SUBSEQUENT THERAPY

1. When erythroderma improves and exfoliation ceases, begin the patient on the Goekerman regimen as described above.
2. Maintenance therapy for psoriasis is often required following resolution of the erythrodermic episode, depending on the morphology of the process.

ALTERNATIVE THERAPY

For patients not responding rapidly to hydration, emollients, and hospitalization, the following alternatives are reasonable:

1. Treat with medium-strength topical corticosteroids in an ointment b.i.d., or in a cream with occlusion if tolerated. Begin the Goekerman regimen following control of erythroderma.
2. Treat with etretinate 0.5–2 mg/kg/day.
3. Treat with methotrexate as described above.
4. Treat with cyclosporin A.

Pustular Psoriasis (Generalized)

INITIAL THERAPY

1. Hospitalize the patient on "bed rest" orders.
2. Assure normal fluid and electrolyte balance.
3. Treat with bland emollients.
4. Start the patient on etretinate 0.25–2 mg/kg/day. Low-dose etretinate (0.25–0.5 mg/kg) is often adequate.

5. Expect significant improvement within 3–7 days.
6. Gradually taper any existing steroid therapy as the patient responds to retinoids. Abrupt discontinuance of existing topical steroid therapy may aggravate pustular flaring.

SUBSEQUENT THERAPY
When pustulation ceases, the following approach is reasonable:

1. Taper retinoids gradually by reducing dose by 0.2–0.3 mg/kg/day weekly unless the disorder recurs.
2. Begin patient on PUVA or the Goekerman regimen. Many patients can be controlled by PUVA or UVB in the absence of etretinate.

ALTERNATIVE THERAPY
1. (Accutane) 13-*cis*-retinoic acid 1–2 mg/kg/day will control pustulation, but is not as effective as etretinate for long-term control.
2. Methotrexate may be used if retinoids are contraindicated.

PITFALLS
1. Do not use systemic corticosteroids; if used as a last resort, pustular flare may follow as steroids are reduced.
2. Antimalarials, lithium, and β-blockers may aggravate pustular flare and should be stopped.

Therapy of Psoriasis of the Palms and Soles (Localized Pustular Psoriasis)

Although this disorder is notoriously difficult to treat, the following alternatives are reasonable and often helpful.

Initial Therapy

The goal of therapy should be control of symptoms and restoration of function. Total clearing of this process is seldom achieved.

1. Soak palms and soles for 15–20 minutes 2–3 ×/day in a tepid tar-containing solution (e.g., Zetar Emulsion) (1–2 tbsps/qt water).
2. After soaking, pat the hands dry and apply a superpotent topical corticosteroid ointment (e.g., Temovate 0.05% ointment or Diprolene 0.05% ointment).

SUBSEQUENT THERAPY

Satisfactory clinical response should be achieved within 14–21 days. Taper therapy to the level needed to maintain control and acceptable to the patient.

ALTERNATIVE THERAPY

If satisfactory control is not achieved, the following alternatives are reasonable:

1. Anthralin.
2. Topical PUVA exposing only the palms and soles.
3. Methotrexate.
4. Etretinate 1–2 mg/kg/day.
5. Cyclosporin A.

Therapy of Psoriasis of the Nails

Although psoriasis-associated nail changes may improve in association with response to therapies such as PUVA, retinoids, methotrexate, or UVB, local nail treatment has been largely ineffective. The following alternatives may be attempted, but they require a highly motivated patient.

1. Apply a high-potency topical steroid to the proximal nail and nailfold and occlude the nails nightly. Therapy may be required for at least 3 months to appreciate any benefit.
2. Inject each nailfold with Kenalog 0.1 cc (5 mg/cc). Repeat therapy after 6–8 weeks as needed if tolerated. This is extremely painful, and is not tolerated by most patients.
3. Remove hypertrophic nails by applying urea 40% ointment to the nails and occluding with plastic and cloth adhesive tape. Keep the nails dry, and remove the dressing after 7 days. The nail can then be easily elevated and removed. After nail removal, apply a superpotent topical steroid to the nail bed and nailfold b.i.d. Regrowth of a possibly (50%) improved nail requires 3–4 months.

BW

148

Pruritic Dermatoses of Pregnancy

Pruritic Urticarial Papules and Plaques of Pregnancy • Papular Dermatitis of Pregnancy

See Chapter 86, Herpes Gestationis, for its management.

Initial Therapy

1. A topical steroid cream applied t.i.d to q.i.d. The strength should be guided guided by the severity of the pruritus.
2. Oral diphenhydramine 25–50 mg t.i.d.

Subsequent Therapy

Only rarely are systemic steroids required in these conditions. Prescribe the minimum effective dose (initially usually 0.5–1 mg/kg q.a.m. tapered to the lowest controlling dose).

Pitfalls

1. Herpes gestationis may initially resemble the pruritic urticarial papules and plaques of pregnancy. A biopsy for direct immunofluorescence may be indicated.
2. Scabies and other insect bites are morphologically similar to the pruritic papular rashes of pregnancy. Look carefully for burrows and take a history of animal exposure.

TB

149

Pyoderma Gangrenosum

Pyoderma gangrenosum (PG) is a syndrome defined by its characteristic morphology. Since PG is associated with several different, underlying disease processes, the choice of therapy will be dictated in many instances by the nature of the provocative condition.

Initial Therapy

This therapy is recommended by Gerald S. Lazarus, M.D. (see, e.g., *Archives of Dermatology* 125:57, 1989).

1. Systemic corticosteroids are the mainstay of treatment for patients with established ulcerations and with multiple lesions. Initial therapy is 60–80 mg/day in divided doses, but if a prompt response is not obtained, much higher doses may be needed. After a response is seen, gradually switch the patient over to a q.d. and then to a q.o.d. regimen before tapering.
2. Local therapy is very effective for early lesions: inject triamicinolone acetonide 10 mg/cc, diluted with lidocaine 1%, directly into inflammatory lesions; inject the same concentration into the rim, using a 30-gauge needle directed from the outside of the rim toward the center. Patients may need to be premedicated with analgesics, such as meperidine plus promethazine, to tolerate injections.
3. Ulcers should be gently debrided with wet soaks, utilizing normal saline, or Domeboro, diluted 1 : 40 with tap water. Apply soaked, fine mesh guaze to the ulcer base, cover with coarse gauze (Kerlex gauze), moisten, and leave for 1 hour. Repeat q.i.d.
4. Between wet dressings, whirlpools may provide additional debridement.
5. Application of silver sulfadiazine (Silvadene) cream between soaks, followed by occlusion with a Telfa pad, may help treat or prevent secondary infections.

Alternative Systemic Therapy

1. According to Lazarus, pulse therapy with suprapharmacologic doses of corticosteroids can produce dramatic involution of lesions. Patients are given methylprednisolone lg/150 ml dextrose in water, infused over 1 hour.

Patients should be monitored during infusions and for 4 hours thereafter, particularly for arrhythmias. Infusions are administered 5 ×/day until a response occurs (usually within 48 hours), then maintained on q.o.d. steroids (prednisone 40–60 mg q.o.d.). Pulse therapy can be repeated every 3–4 weeks, if necessary. *Note:* Patients treated previously or currently with oral steroids, with a history of cardiac arrhythmias, or taking diuretics are not good candidates for pulse therapy because of the risk of additive electrolyte alterations that could lead to arrhythmias (occasionally fatal).

2. Dapsone is effective for PG (as well as for underlying inflammatory bowel disease, when present). After a screen for G6PD deficiency is obtained, therapy is begun at a dose of 50 mg b.i.d. and gradually raised to 300–400 mg/day over a 4-week period. CBC and LFTs must be monitored regularly in patients receiving dapsone.

3. Sulfapyridine is slightly less effective than dapsone for PG, but less toxic, and sulfapyridine is particularly useful for PG associated with inflammatory bowel disease. The initial dose is usually 2 g/day (500 mg q.i.d.), which is then raised to 3 g/day until a good response is achieved. Again, CBC and LFTs must be monitored twice monthly, and patients advised to drink copious amounts of water to minimize drug deposition in their kidneys.

4. Chemotherapeutic agents can be useful as primary or adjunctive therapy of PG. Azathioprine 50–150 mg/day is particularly effective in PG associated with chronic active hepatitis or rheumatoid arthritis. CBC and LFTs are monitored weekly in patients receiving azathioprine (see Appendix 7). Cyclophosphamide may be effective in recalcitrant cases. Doses of up to 2 mg/kg/day are used. Side effects can be severe, especially in patients who are simultaneously receiving systemic steroids (see Appendix 5).

5. Clofazimine 100 mg b.i.d. (see *Dermatologica* 177:232–236, 1988), 2% aqueous sodium chromoglycate, administered as a spray t.i.d. directly to ulcers (see *British Journal of Dermatology* 102:231, 1980), and minocycline have been reported to be of benefit in some cases of PG.

Alternate Topical Therapy

1. Vapor-permeable, hydrophilic membranes, such as Duoderm or Vigilon, stop pain immediately and may hasten re-epithelialization. Dressings should be changed every 24 hrs to avoid bacterial colonization under dressings.

2. Although skin grafts often will "take" in patients receiving systemic steroids, pathergy at the donor site may occur. Hence, grafts should be reserved for large, nonhealing lesions.

3. Hyperbaric oxygen reportedly accelerates healing rates in some patients.

Subsequent Therapy

1. Work-up for an associated disease is mandatory, since control of PG often can be achieved with therapy of the underlying disease process. Inflammatory bowel disease (i.e., both ulcerative colitis and regional enteritis (Crohn's)) is the most common associated illness. Resection of the diseased colon in ulcerative colitis often (but not always) cures the associated PG as well.
2. Healed lesions of PG are extremely susceptible to trauma, and trauma can reactivate previously quiescent lesions. Emollients should be routinely employed, and both elevation and support stockings should be prescribed to minimize venous pooling that can lead to leg ulcers.

Pitfalls

1. Pyoderma gangrenosum-like lesions occur in a host of other diseases, including sarcomas, mycobacterial and other infections, halogenoderma, gummas, Wegener's granulomatosis, and factitia. In new cases, cultures and a wedge biopsy should be obtained for both culture and histopathology from the edge of ulcerating lesions for diagnostic purposes.
2. Pathergy (i.e., appearance of disease in sites of trauma) occurs in about 50% of patients with PG. Hence, aggressive debridement or other manipulations should be avoided.
3. Iodides can aggravate lesions of PG.
4. The pitfalls of systemic steroid therapy are detailed in Appendix 5.
5. The pitfalls of systemic chemotherapeutic agents are detailed in Appendix 7.
6. Sulfones and sulfapyridine can cause a host of toxic and idiosyncratic side effects. Accelerated hemolysis owing to shortened red cell life-span occurs in all patients, but can be life-threatening in patients with G6PD deficiency.

PE

150

Radiation Dermatitis

Radiation dermatitis may be acute or chronic.

ACUTE RADIATION DERMATITIS

The goal of therapy is to reduce erythema, pain, and blistering in this self-limited process. Treatment is symptomatic.

Initial Therapy

1. Elevate the involved part, if possible.
2. Wrap the lesions for 30 minutes t.i.d. to q.i.d. with compress dressings soaked in cool tap water or Burrow's solution, and pat dry.
3. Apply a medium- or high-potency topical corticosteroid cream after soaks.
4. Treat with systemic pain medication as necessary to control pain and discomfort.

Subsequent Therapy

1. Expect resolution of acute inflammation in days to weeks.
2. Desquamation following acute dermatitis may be treated with a bland emollient as necessary.

CHRONIC RADIATION DERMATITIS

The aim of therapy is to prevent malignant degeneration. Associated atrophy, depigmentation, hypopigmentation and telangiectasia are not reversible. Because standard therapy is not defined, alternatives are listed.

Therapeutic Alternatives

1. If possible, carefully excise the area.
2. If actinic keratoses are present, apply 5-fluorouracil as described for treatment of actinic keratosis (see Ch. 5).

3. If malignancy is present, the area must be treated as described for cutaneous malignancies (see Ch. 39).

Pitfalls

1. Additional radiation is absolutely contraindicated.
2. The long-term potential for development of malignancies is real. A non-healing ulcer may result from trauma and slow healing, but may also represent a developing malignancy. All lesions that cannot be practically removed must be closely followed, and all suspicious lesions should be biopsied.

BW

151

Raynaud's Phenomenon/Disease

Peripheral vasospasm can occur as an isolated disease entity (Raynaud's disease) or in association with another disease process, such as collagen vascular diseases (Raynaud's phenomenon). Typically, the digits are involved, but the nose, ears, nipples, and other exposed areas can be affected. The degree of vasospasm is variable, and treatment is mandated by the severity of symptoms.

Initial Therapy (Moderate-to-Severe Cases)

1. Calcium channel blockers, although only introduced relatively recently, are the most effective agents, but are not without side effects (see Pitfalls). Either diltiazepam (Cardizem) 30–60 mg q.i.d. or nifedipine 10–30 mg t.i.d. reportedly are effective, although verapamil does not appear to possess equivalent efficacy. Perform an initial test dose with monitoring of blood pressure in the office, and if no toxicity is observed, therapy can be gradually increased, as needed to control symptoms.
2. Glycerol trinitrate ointment (Nitropaste), applied q.d., may reduce the frequency and severity of attacks. The use of topical vasodilators, if effective, may allow some reduction in the dose of calcium channel blockers or vasodilators.

Alternative Therapy

1. Ketanserin, a recently introduced, specific antagonist of serotonin, has been reported to improve vasospasm and to promote wound healing in Raynaud's phenomenon associated with scleroderma. The dosage employed was 20 mg b.i.d.
2. Vasodilators and/or α-adrenergic blocking agents may increase peripheral blood flow, but do not necessarily prevent Raynaud's phenomenon. Nevertheless, oral phenoxybenzamine 10–60 mg/day, reserpine 0.25 mg b.i.d., prazosin (2–8 mg/day), or oral methyldopa (250 mg b.i.d.) may be useful in selected cases.

Ancillary Therapy

1. Patients should avoid excess exposure to cold. Warm, loose-fitting clothing is preferred, and the entire body must remain warm. Warming involved digits in warm water to terminate vasospastic episodes may decrease the occurrence of ischemic damage.
2. Discontinuation of smoking ameliorates Raynaud's phenomenon. Passive inhalation of smoke also may trigger episodes.
3. Emotional turmoil can aggravate and precipitate Raynaud's phenomenon. Therefore, some patients may be helped by psychotherapy, psychoactive drugs, and/or biofeedback.
4. Trauma should be minimized because of delayed wound-healing and tendency for persistent ulcerations. This may influence choice of, or even dictate changes in, types of occupation.
5. Work-up of Raynaud's phenomenon will reveal an associated systemic disorder in about 40% of cases. Therapy of the underlying disease results in improvement and cure of the associated vasospasm.
6. Debridement, systemic antibiotics, and vapor-permeable membranes may be useful for treating associated ulcerations.
7. Patients can learn to abort a Raynaud's attack by using a whirling arm maneuver. The patient continuously swings his arms in 360° circles in the manner of a softball pitcher. The combination of gravitational and centrifugal forces helps to restore the circulation to the outstretched fingers in 1–2 minutes.

Pitfalls

1. Acral pitting and/or ulcerations may complicate the course of Raynaud's phenomenon in 10%–15% of cases.
2. The associated systemic disease may not surface for years after the initial occurrence of Raynaud's phenomenon, therefore work-ups need to be repeated at regular intervals.
3. Certain drugs, such as ergotamines and β-blockers, can aggravate or

precipitate Raynaud's disease. The possible role of medications in disease activity should be examined carefully.

4. Calcium channel blockers seem to be more beneficial to patients with primary Raynaud's disease as opposed to cases of vasospasm associated with scleroderma or other underlying disorders.

5. Calcium channel blockers can produce toxic side effects, including hypotension, CNS toxicity, aggravation of esophageal reflux, and peripheral edema.

PE

152

Relapsing Polychondritis

Relapsing polychondritis is a multisystem disease that may affect the cartilage of the ear, nose, joints, and respiratory tract; the inner ear; the heart; and the kidney. Therapy is in part directed by the severity of the disease.

Initial Therapy

1. Dapsone 100–200 mg/day initially, then tapered, may be quite beneficial.
2. Systemic corticosteroids are the standard of care and probably should be the initial therapy in those with significant disease. Initial doses of 40–60 mg/day are administered, then tapered.

Alternative Therapy

NSAIDs (e.g., aspirin, indomethacin, or colchicine) are often adequate to control symptoms.

Subsequent Therapy

1. Because the disease may be intermittently active, drug therapy can be tapered and often stopped in controlled cases between episodes.
2. In patients failing to respond to the above therapies, an immunosuppressive agent (e.g., cyclophosphomide, azathioprine, mercaptopurine, or melphalan) may be added to the systemic corticosteroids. These are also useful steroid-sparing agents.

3. Cyclosporin A may be effective in the most severe and difficult to control patients.

Pitfall

Dapsone may cause acute or chronic adverse reactions. A pretherapy screen (including G6PD) must be performed and LFTs and CBC followed during treatment.

TB

153

Reticular Erythematous Mucinosis

Plaque-Like Cutaneous Mucinosis

Initial Therapy

1. Oral hydroxychloroquine (Plaquenil) 200 mg/day for several months.
2. Avoidance of sun exposure to the affected areas, and application of a sunscreen with a SPF of 15 or greater.

Alternative Therapy

Topical corticosteroids usually are of no benefit.

Subsequent Therapy

1. In patients responding to hydroxychloroquine, once clear, the drug may be stopped or the dosage reduced. Relapses may occur and retreatment is advised.
2. In patients failing to respond to hydroxychloroquine 200 mg/day the dosage may be increased to 200 mg b.i.d. or oral chloroquine 250 mg q.d. or b.i.d. may be substituted.

Pitfalls

1. Reticular erythematous mucinosis may resemble subacute cutaneous lupus erythematosus.
2. Antimalarials may cause retinal damage, therefore patients must be screened by an ophthalmologist prior to beginning treatment and at 6-month intervals during therapy. They are contraindicated in pregnancy. Antimalarials may exacerbate psoriasis and porphyria cutanea tarda.

TB

154

Rosacea

Acne Rosacea

Those affected by rosacea may have facial erythema, telangectasia, papules and pustules, or sebaceous hyperplasia of the nose (rhinophyma). Effective medical treatment is available only for the papular and pustular components. The telangectasias and rhinophyma may be surgically treated (see below), but only after the patient has had adequate medical therapy. Mild to moderate improvement of the erythema may occur during therapy.

Initial Therapy

1. Stop all topical corticosteroids stronger than hydrocortisone 1%. If the patient has been using them, anticipate a flare when they are discontinued.
2. Advise the patient to avoid sunexposure, wear a hat, and use a non-comedogenic sunscreen (Ti screen, Presun 29) every morning.
3. Advise reduction or elimination of alcohol ingestion.
4. Prescribe oral tetracycline 250–500 mg b.i.d. depending on the severity of the rosacea.
5. Metronidazole 250 mg b.i.d. is as effective as tetracycline. Topical metronidazole 0.75% gel b.i.d. is available and often adequate for patients previously requiring oral antibiotics.

Alternative Therapy

1. Cases of mild rosacea may be controlled with topical antibiotics (erythromycin 2% solution, clindamycin 1%, Meclan Cr).

2. Benzoyl peroxide 2.5% in a water-based gel on alternate nights may be adjunctively useful.
3. For the pregnant patient topical erythromycin 2% solution or oral erythromycin 250–500 mg b.i.d. may be used.

Subsequent Therapy

Most patients with rosacea (except those in whom the rosacea was induced or exacerbated by topical steroids) will require some form of maintenance therapy.

INITIALLY IMPROVED

1. Taper the oral or topical therapy by 50% each month until the patient begins to break through. Often very low dose tetracycline (e.g., 250 mg 2×/week) will maintain patients.
2. Cases controlled with oral agents may occasionally require only topical antibiotics for maintenance.

INITIALLY UNIMPROVED

1. Increase the tetracycline dosage to 1–2 g/day.
2. Oral metronidazole 250 mg b.i.d.; or topical 0.75% gel b.i.d.
3. Oral minocycline 100 mg q.d. to b.i.d. will occasionally control cases failing to respond to oral tetracycline.
4. 13-*cis* retinoic acid (Accutane) in low doses (10–40 mg/day) will usually improve rosacea. The safety of chronic usage at these doses is unknown. This therapy should be avoided in the female patient with childbearing potential.

Pitfalls

1. Tetracycline, minocycline, and 13-*cis* retinoic acid are contraindicated in pregnancy. Adequately documented contraception, a negative pregnancy test, and extensive counselling are required before a woman of childbearing potential is administered one of these agents.
2. Patients taking oral metronidazole may develop a disulfiram reaction when ingesting alcohol.
3. Patients whose rosacea is induced or exacerbated by topical steroids may suffer a severe flare after they discontinue the steroid. The care provider must warn the patient of this, and explain that although the topical steroid appears to improve the rosacea, it is actually causing it as well.
4. Patients with rosacea have sensitive skin in general and tolerate topical irritants poorly. Usually tretinoin (Retin-A) or high concentrations of benzoyl peroxide are not recommended.

5. The use of 13-*cis* retinoic acid is best prescribed by those physicians with experience with this agent and its multitudinous side effects. Because it may raise serum cholesterol and triglycerides and reduce high-density lipoproteins it is relatively contraindicated in those with lipid abnormalities, diabetes, or other atherosclerotic vascular disease.

Surgical Treatment

TELANGECTASIAS AND ERYTHEMA

1. Telangectasias may be treated with bipolar electrosurgery.
2. Laser therapy, especially with a pulse dye laser, may be used for both the persistent erythema and the telangectasias.

RHINOPHYMA

Surgical procedures for the reduction of rhinophyma are uniformly successful, have a low complication rate, and give high patient satisfaction. Patients who are psychologically distressed by their appearance should be encouraged to seek dermatologic surgery consultation.

1. Electrosurgical sculpturing of the rhinophymatous nose gives excellent results, is fast, and is almost bloodless. It is equivalent to laser therapy, although it may be more likely to scar.
2. A laser may also be used for the treatment of rhinophyma, although it is more costly and more time-consuming than electrosurgical treatment.
3. Cold-steel surgery and dermabrasion are also effective, but they are more difficult owing to the vascularity of the nose.

TB

155

Sarcoidosis

The course of sarcoidosis ranges from acute episodes followed by early spontaneous remissions, as in hilar adenopathy-erythema nodosum syndrome, to chronic, unremitting disease accompanied by one or more of the following: restrictive pulmonary disease, uveitis, hepatosplenomegaly, and disfiguring skin lesions. Patients with multisystem disease are best managed by a team of appropriate specialists.

DISFIGURING SKIN LESIONS ALONE

Initial Therapy

1. Topical steroids under occlusion: Apply pieces of a steroid-impregnated flurandrenolide tape (Cordran) over lesions q.h.s. For acral lesions apply any intermediate-potency steroid in a cream formulation, and then occlude with either plastic wrap or plastic bag q.h.s.
2. Intralesional steroids: Inject triamcinolone acetonide (Kenalog) 10 mg/cc directly into lesions monthly for several months.
3. For treatment of erythema nodosum, see Chapter 63.

Alternate Therapy

1. Antimalarials: Hydroxychlorquine (Plaquenil) 200 mg b.i.d. or chloroquine 250 mg b.i.d. for 2 weeks, followed by a 50% reduction of the dose is usually effective, but should be discontinued after 6 months to decrease the likelihood of ocular side effects.
2. Systemic steroids: Administer initially at a dose of 40 mg q.a.m. with gradual tapering over several months to 15–20 mg/day. Patients often can be maintained on q.o.d. therapy indefinitely at relatively low doses (e.g., 20 mg. q.o.d. in the morning).
3. Certain immunosuppressive chemotherapeutic agents (e.g., azathioprine, chlorambucil) can produce involution of lesions.
4. The systemic retinoids etretinate and acitretin have reportedly improved skin lesions in some patients. If steroids and antimalarials are not helpful, therapy can be begun at a dose of 1–2 mg/kg/day (usually 25 mg t.i.d.) × 6–8 weeks, with gradual tapering as improvement occurs (see Appendix 6 for precautions and potential pitfalls of systemic retinoid therapy).

MULTISYSTEM DISEASE

Initial Therapy

Prescribe systemic steroids and/or chemotherapeutic agents at the doses indicated above, with additional, specific ophthalmologic and pulmonary therapy directed by appropriate specialists.

Pitfalls

The pitfalls of occlusive and intralesional steroids, sytemic steroids, and immunosuppressive agents are described in Appendices 5–7, and those of antimalarials are described in Chapter 48.

PE

156

Scabies

Initial Therapy

1. For adults (except pregnant women), and children over 5 years: Prescribe lindane lotion to be applied from the neck to the tips of the toes and fingers and left on for 12 hours. If the head and neck are involved, treat it as well. The lotion is massaged under *trimmed* fingernails.
2. For children between 1 and 6 years of age: Prescribe crotamiton 10% lotion to be applied from the neck to the tips of the toes and fingers and left on for 24 hours, and repeated the next 24 hours. If the head and neck are involved, treat them and the scalp as well. The safety of this agent in pregnancy and infants is not established.
3. For babies under 1 year of age, pregnant women, or the severely malnourished: Prescribe applications of precipitated sulfur 6% in petrolatum to be left on for 24 hours a day for 2–3 days. The head, neck, and scalp of babies are commonly infected and require treatment. The efficacy of this therapy has been questioned by some experts.
4. Treat all household members and sexual contacts at the same time.
5. All clothing and bedding used prior to treatment should be washed and dried in a dryer, if possible. Nonwashable clothing and bedding should be sealed in a plastic bag for 2 weeks, or dry cleaned.
6. For those with dermatitis a medium-potency topical steroid applied b.i.d. to q.i.d. and oral antihistamines should be used as well.
7. For those with secondary infection give oral antistaphylococcal antibiotics for 1 week.

Alternative Therapy

Crotamiton 10% lotion may be used for two consecutive 24-hour periods. Five days of consecutive therapy may be more effective than shorter courses and should be considered in severe cases.

Subsequent Therapy

PATIENT IMPROVED

1. In those with initial heavy infestations, lindane may be repeated *after 1 week.* Persons who have thick or crusted lesions frequently require a repeat course of treatment.

2. After the initial antiscabetic treatment, prescribe medium-potency steroids to be applied b.i.d. to t.i.d. for those with dermatitis.
3. Oral antihistamines may be necessary for days to weeks to help control persistent pruritus.
4. Scabetic nodules of the penis, axillary lines, and periumbilical area may persist for up to 1 year. Potent topical steroids, tar gels, or dilute intralesional steroid injections (2.0 mg/cc) may be required to eradicate them.

PATIENT NOT IMPROVED

1. Repeat skin examination and scrapings are indicated in those in whom the dermatitis does not improve within 7–10 days. Lindane therapy is repeated.
2. If initial therapy with crotamiton or precipitated sulfur is not effective, lindane lotion may be used. Carefully inform the patients of potential side effects and stress the importance of correct application.
3. Treat all household and sexual contacts.

Pitfalls

1. The major failure in managing scabies is not confirming the diagnosis by skin scrapings prior to treatment. Subsequent therapy must often be empiric. Since many persons must often be treated, undocumented diagnosis should be avoided.
2. Most therapeutic failures are related to improper use of the topical agents. The topical scabicides must be applied *to the whole cutaneous surface* (below the neck except in young children and those with head and neck lesions). Antiscabetic medications are *never* applied to the lesions only. Care must be taken to apply the topicals carefully between the fingers and toes, and under the fingernails, which should be trimmed short. If hands are washed during the treatment period, the medication must be reapplied.
3. Another major reason treatment fails is that all affected persons are not treated *at the same time*. All family members, *even if they don't itch*, must be treated. In households where there are babies, this includes babysitters and occasional visitors who have held the baby. Sexual contacts must also be treated. Infested persons may not itch for 4–6 weeks after acquiring infection, yet may infect others.
4. Lindane toxicity occurs very rarely if it is used correctly. To avoid toxicity:
   a. Use only when indicated.
   b. Do not bathe before applying.
   c. Do not repeat treatment more often than once weekly.
5. The safety of crotamiton in pregnancy and childhood is not established. It

has been used less than lindane, which is available without a prescription in Canada. For this reason certain experts prescribe lindane with careful patient instruction for all scabies patients owing to its proven efficacy. Patient education and informed consent are essential.

6. For the thumbsucking infant using lindane, treat overnight and occlude the sucked digit during treatment with a sock.

7. Breast-feeding mothers may store milk to feed the infant and not breast feed for several days after they use lindane. Alternatively, they may use 6% precipitated sulfur.

8. Crotamiton may fail in short courses (24–48 hours) but be effective in longer courses (i.e., 5 consecutive days).

TB

157

Scleroderma

Progressive Systemic Sclerosis

Scleroderma may be localized (morphea; see Ch. 113) or generalized/systemic (progressive systemic sclerosis (PSS)). Although occasionally patients with localized scleroderna can develop multiple lesions, systemic involvement usually does not occur. Therapy of the various forms of scleroderma is directed toward relief of symptoms as they appear. The management of Raynaud's phenomenon and other vasospastic complications is outlined in Chapter 151. Patients with systemic sclerosis are best managed by a team of specialists; therefore, these recommendations primarily address the management of cutaneous disease.

Initial Therapy

1. Prednisone 40–60 mg/day in divided doses for 1 month, followed by tapering to 20 mg/day for 2 months. Discontinue steroids after 3 months. Steroids are used alone or with plasmapheresis.

2. Recent studies suggest that plasmapheresis with systemic steroids may be

indicated for the accelerated phase of PSS (plasmapheresis alone, however, has not been proven to be helpful).

Alternate Therapy

1. Chemotherapeutic agents: Azathioprine (Imuran) 100–200 mg/day has been used in scleroderma with variable results. The alkylating agents, chlorambucil and cyclophosphamide, also have been reported to benefit some patients. Chemotherapeutic agents also can be combined with plasmapheresis and/or steroids.
2. D-penicillamine, an inhibitor of collagen synthesis, has reportedly softened sclerosis, slowed visceral involvement, and improved overall prognosis in some studies. Begin with a dose of 250 mg/day for 1 month, then increase first to 500 mg/day for 1 month, and then change to a maintenance dose of 750 mg/day as tolerated.
3. Cyclofenil, a derivative of stilbestrol that decreases proteoglycan synthesis, may improve mobility and provide subjective relief. The dose is 300 mg/day for 21 consecutive days each month.

Pitfalls

1. Systemic sclerosis progresses to an accelerated, malignant phase, characterized by progressive renal failure and severe hypertension. Nephrectomy may be life-saving in such cases.
2. Most patients with systemic sclerosis have esophageal involvement, characterized by esophagitis and/or dysphagia, that responds to a standard peptic-ulcer regimen (i.e., H_2 blockers, frequent small feedings, and antacids).
3. Calcinosis cutis develops in about 10% of patients, usually over joints and forearms. Ulceration and/or secondary infection can result, and should be treated with surgical debridement, compresses, and systemic antibiotics. Calcium chelating agents do not appear to be helpful.
4. D-penicillamine exhibits frequent, serious side effects, including bone marrow suppression, nephrotoxicity, GI distress, severe skin reactions (including lupus erythematosus and pemphigus vulgaris-like reactions), and a toxic myasthenia syndrome. Pyridoxine vitamin and mineral supplementation may reduce GI and myasthenic side effects. Persistent bone marrow suppression and proteinuria (monitor CBC and urinalysis every 2 weeks for the first 6 months) mandate discontinuation of drug. However, most side effects become minimal after several months of therapy.
5. For side effects of systemic and topical steroids, see Appendices 3 and 5.
6. For side effects of chemotherapeutic agents, see Appendix 7.

PE

158

Seborrheic Dermatitis

At present there is controversy about the etiology of seborrheic dermatitis, with some believing that a yeast organism, *P. orbiculare*, is the primary cause, while others believe that this organism is only a secondary colonizer. Seborrheic dermatitis can be limited to the scalp, but it also can involve the face, any hairy or intertriginous area, and rarely can even progress to a generalized erythroderma. Seborrheic dermatitis often coexists and/or overlaps with other diseases, including psoriasis (sebopsoriasis), acne rosacea, and acne vulgaris. In this chapter, attention is focused on the management of the seborrheic process only.

Initial Therapy

SCALP

1. For moderate seborrheic dermatitis, prescribe an intermediate-potency steroid-containing solution (e.g., triamcinolone acetonide 0.1% in propylene glycol, fluocinonide 0.05% (Lidex), or betamethasone diproprionate 0.05% (Diprosone) solution) to be applied q.h.s. For best and most economical results, the solution should be streaked in three parallel rows (about 4–5 drops in each row), and massaged into the scalp.
2. For severe seborrheic dermatitis, the efficacy of the topical steroid can be enhanced by wearing an air-tight, plastic shower cap overnight after steroid application.
3. In all cases of seborrheic dermatitis, a cosmetically acceptable tar-containing shampoo (e.g., DHS-T, Vanseb-T, T/Gel, Ionil-T) should be used q.d. Since these preparations may produce some dryness of the hair, or impart a slight odor, patients may follow medicated shampoo treatments with a conditioner or cream rinse.

BODY

Seborrheic dermatitis of nonscalp regions is extremely steroid-responsive, and therefore potent fluorinated steroids need not be used. Moreover, since the face and body folds are often involved, prescribe a nonfluorinated (nonatrophogenic) steroid (e.g., desonide 0.5% (Tridesilon) or hydrocortisone 2.5% cream (Hytone)) to be applied b.i.d. or t.i.d.

Ancillary Therapy for More Recalcitrant Cases

1. Baker's P&S or T/Gel lotion can be applied q.h.s. along with steroid solution to further loosen adherent scale.
2. The possibility of a pathogenic yeast infection should be considered in resistent cases, and topical ketoconazole cream q.h.s. to scalp and other affected areas for 21 days can be tried (in conjunction with other ongoing topical therapy).

Subsequent Therapy

1. After initial treatment improvement, the goals of therapy are to reduce reliance on topical steroids, and to maintain progress gained with medicated shampoos. Even when nonscalp areas are involved, ongoing therapy of scalp alone often will maintain progress, suggesting that "seeding" downward may be responsible for more widespread disease. By 2–4 weeks, patients often can be weaned off topical steroids, and maintained on regular shampooing with medicated shampoos alone.
2. Seborrheic dermatitis can exacerbate and/or coexist with acne vulgaris and acne rosacea, for which additional therapy may be indicated (see Chs. 2 and 154, respectively).
3. In the rare exfoliative erythroderma, ascribable to seborrheic dermatitis, underlying sepsis should be ruled out.

Pitfalls

1. In recalcitrant cases rule out psoriasis or tinea capitis.
2. In addition to the coexisting conditions described above, a seborrheic dermatitis-like picture can be the presenting feature of all forms of histiocytosis X syndromes and other rare inherited or congenital disorders (e.g., Hailey-Hailey disease, complement deficiencies).
3. Seborrheic dermatitis tends to recur and relapse repeatedly; therefore, therapy with medicated shampoos (and often intermittent topical steroids as well) may need to be continued indefinitely.
4. Potent, topical, fluorinated steroids are often prescribed by nondermatologists for the facial rash of seborrheic dermatitis. This is a common cause of steroid-induced rosacea. Such patients need to be weaned off potent steroids with a combination of nonfluorinated preparations (e.g., desonide cream), and often oral tetracycline (250 mg t.i.d. for 30 days, followed by tapering over an additional 30–60 days). Finally, such patients may need therapy of the underlying seborrheic dermatitis, when this complication has subsided.

5. Seborrheic dermatitis after infancy and before adolescence is rare (owing to inactivity of sebaceous glands). In contrast, tinea capitis is common in this age group. The presence of various degrees of hair loss is suggestive of tinea capitis. A fungal culture and/or scraping should be taken to exclude tinea in this age group before using corticosteroids on the scalp.

PE

159

Seborrheic Keratosis

Initial Therapy

1. Light cryotherapy.
2. With or without local anesthesia, removal with a sharp curette; light cautery of the base may be necessary for hemostasis.

Subsequent Therapy

Lesions partly removed by one application of cryotherapy may be frozen again after 3–4 weeks.

Pitfalls

1. Seborrheic keratoses are pigmented lesions. If there is any doubt as to the diagnosis, referral or a biopsy is essential.
2. Cryotherapy in persons of moderate to dark complexion may lead to permanent hypopigmentation.
3. Overaggressive cryotherapy or cautery may cause scarring.
4. Persistent lesions may be removed by shave or excisional biopsy.

TB

160

Solar Urticaria

In this uncommon disorder, exposure to light causes rapid urticaria only in the light-exposed skin. If large areas of skin are exposed, hypotension and bronchospasm may be induced. Although this disorder has been subclassified into six types, the following practical approach is reasonable for most patients. The goal of therapy is to control symptoms so the patient can tolerate exposure to light.

Initial Therapy

1. Treat with an H_1-blocking antihistamine. Begin with hydroxyzine (Atarax) 25–50 mg q.i.d. or the nonsedating antihistamine astemizole (Hismanal) 10-30 mg q.d. and cyproheptadine 4 mg q.i.d. Increase the antihistamine dose weekly until the process is controlled or side effects are not tolerated. Other H_1 antagonists (e.g., the nonsedating antihistamine Seldane) may be used with or without cyproheptadine.
2. Recommend regular applications of a sun screen that effectively blocks both UVA and UVB to light-exposed skin (e.g, Photoplex and SolBar 50 claim to be effective against wavelengths up to 370 nm).
3. Instruct the patient to avoid unnecessary exposure to sunlight; a hat should be worn and the skin covered with tightly woven natural-fiber clothing before sun exposure (loose-weave and synthetic fibers may allow passage of some sunlight to the skin).

Subsequent Therapy

Therapy may be required for years, but requirements may vary throughout the year, with some patients requiring little or no treatment during winter months.

Alternative Therapy

For patients who do not respond to the above therapy:

1. Desensitize with UVA light. Treat with suburticarial doses of UVA light 3 ×/week, increasing exposure by 0.5 J/cm^2 each treatment. If symptoms

275

are induced, hold exposure constant. If clinical control is attained, reduce treatment to the exposure level necessary to maintain a satisfactory response.
2. Desensitize with PUVA. Individuals who do not respond to UVA alone may respond to PUVA. Two hours after treatment with oral methoxsalen (psoralen) (0.6 mg/kg), expose the patient to suburticarial doses of UVA. Treat 3 ×/week while gradually increasing UVA exposure over an 8-week period. Assiduously protect the patient's eyes and skin from sun exposure while methoxsalen is present in the blood (i.e., during and following treatment), and be alert to PUVA side effects as detailed in Chapter 147, Psoriasis.

Pitfalls

1. Patients who do not respond to initial therapy may have erythropoietic protoporphyria (type VI solar urticaria). These individuals should be treated with oral β-carotene.
2. Care must be taken to avoid generalized urticaria and hypotension during desensitization. Determine the suburticarial dose of light prior to treatment by exposing limited areas of skin to UVA until urticaria is induced, then desensitize with 50%–60% of this UVA dose.

BW

161

Spider Bites

Brown Recluse • Black Widow • *Loxoceles* • *Lactrodectus*

BROWN RECLUSE SPIDER (*LOXOCELES RECLUSA*)

Toxins of *Loxoceles* spiders are largely cytotoxic (dermonecrotic). Local reactions are most common, but generalized reactions can occur. Ninety percent of bites are not severe and special treatment is not required. Lesions developing bullae, marked erythema, pain, or ischemia in the first 6–8 hours require more aggressive therapy. Some of these bites may progress to large (up to 20 cm) necrotic ulcers that may take weeks to months to heal.

Initial Therapy

1. Elevate and rest the bitten area. Apply ice, *not* heat.
2. Give analgesics as needed for pain. *Aspirin* is indicated if tolerated, as it is also associated with an improved outcome.
3. Dapsone in doses from 50 to 200 mg/day, depending on the severity of the local reaction, may prevent progression and reduce morbidity.
4. The use of *systemic steroids* is controversial. If used, they should be given early (within 6–8 hours of the bite), and in full doses (i.e., 1 mg/kg/day initially), and tapered over 10–14 days. Steroids should be used to treat all systemic reactions (i.e., hemolysis, thrombocytopenia, convulsions).
5. Early surgery (within 3–4 hours of the bite) is recommended by some authorities, but is controversial. Removal of the lesion may ameliorate systemic symptoms. Dapsone was superior to primary excision in recent reviews, and except in unusual circumstances, surgery should be delayed.
6. Secondary infection almost inevitably occurs. Appropriate antibiotic coverage for *S. aureus* and group A streptococcus is required.

Subsequent Therapy

1. Once the eschar forms, the affected area may be excised surgically. Grafting may be required, but the success rate is low.
2. The patient should be educated on the *L. reclusa* habitat (old clothes, junk- and woodpiles). These areas should be fumigated.

BLACK WIDOW SPIDER (*LACTRODECTUS MACTANS*)

Local reaction is not usually a problem. The venom contains components that are neurotoxic. Muscle spasm, including a board-like abdomen suggesting an acute abdominal emergency, may occur.

Initial Therapy

1. Elevate, rest, and apply cool compresses to the area of the bite. (The patient may not know the site of the bite.)

2. The best and most specific treatment is intramuscular or intravenous antivenin (Lyovac), given exactly as directed by the package insert (2.5 ml).
3. For relief of muscle pain or spasms:
   a. Intravenous calcium gluconate 10 ml of 10% solution, and/or
   b. Intravenous benzodiazepines (e.g., diazepam) or methocarbamol, and/or
   c. Judicious use of morphine sulfate.

Subsequent Therapy

1. Calcium gluconate gives relief for 1–4 hours only, so doses may need to be repeated.
2. A methocarbamol drip, or oral methocarbamol may be used for the 8–36-hour period required for muscle spasms to resolve.
3. The patient should be educated on the *L. mactans* habitat (eaves, privies). These areas should be fumigated.

Pitfalls

1. Calcium gluconate infusions should be given only when the patient's heart rate and rhythm are being monitored.
2. Antivenin is a horse serum-derived product. Immediate (anaphylaxis) and delayed (serum sickness) allergic responses can occur. Skin and conjunctival testing should be performed before giving the antivenin, to rule out immediate hypersensitivity. Due to the small volume given, serum sickness is unlikely to occur.

TB

162

Sporotrichosis

The usual reservoir for sporotrichosis is decaying vegetation or sphagnum moss. Disease follows accidental inoculation of the organism by thorns or splinters. Cats also get sporotrichosis, and can transmit to man. Although pulmonary and disseminated (rare) forms exist, therapeutic guidelines provided are for the chronic lymphocutaneous form of the disease.

Initial Therapy

Saturated solution of potassium iodide (SSKI) is the preferred therapy. Begin with 10 drops (1 g/ml) t.i.d. after meals until the disease is cleared. If the response is poor, push SSKI to the maximum tolerated dose. Significant clearing should occur within 4–6 weeks. If iodism occurs (see Pitfalls), stop treatment for 2–3 days, and resume therapy at a somewhat lower dose.

Alternative Therapy

1. Amphotericin B (Fungizone) should be administered intravenously to cases unresponsive to SSKI (see Ch. 31, Coccidioidomycosis, for guidelines).
2. Oral ketoconozole (Nizonal) has been reported to be helpful in a few cases.

Pitfalls

1. The lymphangitic lesions of sporotrichosis must be differentiated from some types of atypical mycobacterial and nocardial infection. Tularemia and staphylococcal lymphangitis can present with clinically similar lesions, but patients are usually febrile.
2. As with all systemic mycoses, erythema nodosum may occur.
3. Iodism is a universal, dose-related concomitant of SSKI therapy. Symptoms include coryza, rhinorrhea, nausea, and a toxic iododerma. Therapy should be adjusted according to drug tolerance.
4. For side effects of amphotericin B, see Ch. 31, Coccidioidomycosis.

PE

163

Squamous Cell Carcinoma

Squamous cell carcinoma of the skin can be divided into two groups: those lesions with a low risk for metastases, and those with a higher risk for metastases. Low-risk lesions are those arising from actinic keratoses (not of the lower lip) in immunocompetent persons. Higher-risk lesions are those occurring in sites of chronic ulceration, following radiation therapy, on the lower lip or temple, and in the immunosuppressed (especially the renal transplant patient). Higher-risk lesions should be managed only by those with considerable expertise in the evaluation and management of cutaneous malignancy, and is not further discussed.

Initial Therapy

1. Surgical excision with pathologic evaluation of the margins for adequacy of resection is the optimum treatment.
2. Careful palpation before surgery of lymph nodes draining the affected site is required.
3. Stress sun protection (sunscreens and hats), and avoidance of unnecessary sun exposure.

Alternative Therapy

1. Destructive measures (curettage and desiccation or cryotherapy) may also be curative, but do not provide margins for pathologic confirmation of adequacy of resection.
2. For the frail or for lesions in difficult locations, radiation therapy is excellent.

Subsequent Therapy

Periodic examination of the surgery site, draining lymph nodes, and the rest of the patient's exposed skin should be performed.

Pitfalls

1. Failure to recognize higher-risk lesions and treat them adequately can lead to local recurrence or metastases.

2. A complete skin examination should be performed on at least the initial visit in the patient with cutaneous squamous cell carcinoma.

TB

164

Staphylococcal Scalded Skin Syndrome

Staphylococcal scalded skin snydrome (SSSS) is a disease primarily of infants and young children that manifests as a localized process (see Ch. 95, Impetigo); a *forme fruste*, scarlatiniform eruption that never progresses to full-blown necrolysis; a generalized process, characterized by sterile bullae and an occult focus of infection; or a generalized form of bullous impetigo, with spread of infected, bullous lesions to contiguous sites of infection.

The bullous lesions in all forms of SSSS are due to elaboration of epidermolytic toxin by resident pathogenic staphylococci (usually group II, phage type 55 or 71). Because toxic epidermal necrolysis (TEN) owing to drugs or graft vs. host disease also can occur in the pediatric age group, the diagnosis needs to be definitively established by culture, histology, and/or exfoliative cytology. Even though antibiotic therapy has not been shown to influence the outcome of SSSS, aggressive therapy is indicated both to prevent complications and to interrupt epidemics.

Initial Therapy

In this chapter antibiotic doses are given in mg/kg/day, as most patients are infants.

1. For generalized forms of SSSS: Intravenous nafcillin or methicillin 100 mg/kg/day in q.6.h. divided for 48 hours, followed by oral dicloxacillin 50 mg/kg/day for 10 days.

2. Alternative Initial Therapy (in penicillin-allergic individuals): After an initial test dose to ensure non-cross-reactivity, intravenous cephalexin 25 mg/kg/day in q.6.h. divided doses for 48 hours, followed by oral cephalexin 15 mg/kg/day for a total of 10 days, or intravenous vancomycin 9 mg/kg/day in q.6.h. divided doses for 48 hours, followed by oral sulfamethoxasole-trimethoprim (Bactrim or Septra DS) 1 tablet b.i.d.; oral rifampicin 1 mg/kg/day; or oral clindamycin 8 mg/kg/day. Therapy with alternative agents should be guided by antibiotic susceptibility screening.
3. For localized forms (and scarlatiniform eruption), oral dicloxacillin 50 mg/kg/day in individual q.i.d. doses for 10 days.

Alternative Therapy in Penicillin-Allergic Individuals

Oral cephalexin 15 mg/kg/day in divided doses (monitor for possible penicillin-cross reactivity), oral rifampicin 1mg/kg/day for 10 days, or oral clindamycin 8 mg/kg/day for 10 days.

1. Gentle debridement of necrotic, nonadherent bullae daily.
2. Applications of an antibiotic ointment (e.g., silver sulfadiazine (Silvadene) or mupirocin (Bactroban)) to denuded areas b.i.d. after debridement and soaks.
3. Monitor fluid and electrolyte status. Although the high epidermal cleavage plane in SSSS results in rapid regeneration of an effective cutaneous barrier (1–2 days), because of their high surface area to volume ratio, infants are at greater risk for dehydration. Thus, until healing is underway (in approximately 48 hours), monitor weight, intake/output, and blood pressure carefully.

Subsequent Management

1. Reverse isolation precautions should be practiced. SSSS tends to spread in an epidemic fashion through newborn nurseries and infant in-patient wards.
2. Although the skin lesions are largely self-healing, sepsis with arthritis, endocarditis, and osteomyelitis all have been noted in SSSS patients. Moreover, referred patients often have been treated incorrectly with systemic steroids, because of the still widespread belief that TEN and SSSS are related. Prior administration of steroids greatly increases the risk of septic complications and can prolong the course.

Pitfalls

1. The highly contagious nature of the causative staphylococci can result in miniepidemics both within and outside of the hospital. Thus, a search for both symptomatic and asymptomatic carriers in families, nursing personnel, or other in-patients is mandatory. Nasal carriage is most common; hence, empiric therapy (topical antibacterial swabs and bathing with antibacterial cleansers) is advisable for suspected carriers; documented carriers also should receive a short course of therapy with oral dicloxacillin, 250 mg q.i.d. for 7 days for adults, plus rifampicin, 300 mg b.i.d.
2. Concomitant steroid therapy can prolong the course and increase risk of complications (see above), and is therefore contraindicated.
3. Sulfamylon should be avoided if any question of drug-induced TEN exists, and serum osmolarity should be monitored in infants treated with silver sulfadiazine because of the risk of systemic absorption of propylene glycol.

165

Stasis Dermatitis and Stasis Ulcer

Stasis dermatitis and ulcers are complications of chronic venous insufficiency and resultant edema of the lower extremity.

STASIS DERMATITIS

Initial Therapy

1. Control of edema is mandatory!
   a. Elevate the lower extremity by raising the foot of the bed; elevate the foot above the knee and hip while sitting. When possible, encourage lower-extremity muscle-pump activity by walking; discourage standing, but encourage "toe-risers" when standing is unavoidable;

  b. Employ elastic stockings of at least mid-thigh length to firmly but gently compress the extremity.
2. Prescribe a medium-potency topical corticosteroid cream b.i.d. to dermatitic skin. Compression stockings may be worn after steroid application. Expect resolution of dermatitis in 7–14 days.
3. If cellulitis is present, hospitalize the patient, culture the blood, and treat with intravenous antibiotics to provide coverage for staphylococcal and streptococcal infection.

Subsequent Therapy

1. Continue compression and elevation therapy.
2. Xerosis and scaling frequently follow dermatitis; apply an emollient regularly as-needed (Eucerin is excellent, but may not be well tolerated with elastic support stockings; other mineral oil-based emollients may be satisfactory).

Alternative Therapy

Control of edema by simple physical measures may not be possible in some individuals. For such patients consider:

1. A low-salt diet.
2. Use of a diuretic.

Pitfalls

1. Peripheral edema may be caused by mechanisms other than venous insufficiency. Consider congestive heart failure, lymphatic obstruction (filariasis, etc.) or fibrosis, and myxedema, as well as other causes of dermal deposition.
2. Dermatitis may result from chemical contact rather than stasis. Patients may have used topical preparations containing sensitizers such as lanolin, parabens, ethylenediamine, neomycin, or other sensitizers. An adequate history should confirm or eliminate this possibility.

STASIS ULCER

Stasis ulcers frequently occur, and may be successfully treated by numerous techniques. The following approach is not exhaustive but seems reasonable.

Initial Therapy

1. Control edema and dermatitis as described above. Ulcers will not respond to any program in the presence of edema.
2. Culture the ulcer and treat the surrounding cellulitis with an antibiotic appropriate for the isolated pathogens.
3. Debride the ulcer(s).
4. To reduce the bacterial population of the ulcer base apply bacitracin ointment, and cover with a semiocclusive dressing (e.g., Duoderm or Restore) for 7 days.
5. On a weekly basis, measure the ulcer (to document change) and reapply dressings.

Subsequent Therapy

After the ulcer heals, carefully continue the program of edema control.

Alternative Therapy

Many alternatives have been described; the following is a partial but useful list.

1. Apply Unna Boot(s) weekly instead of a semiocclusive dressing.
2. Wet-to-dry dressings may be helpful for debridement, but are difficult to accomplish in the home setting.
3. For difficult ulcers, hospitalize the patient for control of edema, infection, debridement, and proper care of difficult ulcers.

Pitfalls

A nonhealing ulcer may be cutaneous carcinoma (basal cell, squamous cell).

BW

166

Subcorneal Pustular Dermatosis

Sneddon-Wilkinson Syndrome

Initial Therapy

1. Begin treatment of adults with oral dapsone 100 mg/day, increasing by 50 mg/week until the patient responds; most patients respond to 100–150 mg/day, but some will require up to 300 mg/day.
2. Obtain the following laboratory data before treatment: G6PD level, CBC with differential, creatinine, BUN, LFT, and urinalysis.
3. Dapsone-caused hemolysis is dose dependent; check the CBC weekly until a stable dose is established.

Subsequent Therapy

1. When remission occurs, reduce dapsone in 25–50-mg increments each week until the lowest effective maintenance dose is reached. Some patients may be weaned from dapsone, but others will require chronic, long-term maintenance.
2. Check LFTs, creatinine, BUN, and urinalysis every 3 weeks initially, and then every 3 months during maintenance therapy.

Alternative Therapy

1. Treat with sulfapyridine 500 mg q.i.d. and expect improvement within 7–14 days. If clinical response is inadequate, increase the dose by 1 g each week; up to 6 g/day may be required for control. When control is attained, gradually decrease the dose to the lowest amount necessary to maintain clinical response.
2. High-potency topical corticosteroids may be of limited benefit in initial attempts to control pustulation.
3. Etretinate 0.5–1.0 mg/kg/day is an additional alternative. Expect a therapeutic response within 2–4 weeks.

Pitfalls

1. Hemolysis occurs regularly during dapsone or sulfapyridine therapy. A baseline CBC and G6PD are required. Monitor the CBC every 2 weeks when dosage is being increased, and every 1–3 months after the dosage has been stabilized.
2. Dapsone will induce methemoglobinemia, and may cause clinically important cyanosis and complaints of shortness of breath. Methemoglobinemia may be treated with ascorbic acid 200 mg/day (see Ch. 84, Hansen's disease, for complete discussion of pitfalls associated with dapsone therapy).
3. Sneddon-Wilkinson pustular dermatosis may be confused with other pustular disorders, including psoriasis. Lack of response to dapsone or sulfapyridine suggests improper diagnosis. Skin biopsy and consultation with another dermatologist may aid in this differential diagnosis.
4. Other dapsone side effects may include cutaneous eruption, hypersensitivity syndrome (infectious mononucleosis), psychosis, nausea, vomiting, peripheral neuropathy, vertigo, blurred vision, tinnitus, insomnia, headaches, tachycardia, albuminuria, hypoalbuminemia, renal papillary necrosis, cholestasis, hepatitis, and male infertility.

BW

167

Sweet Syndrome

Acute Febrile Neutrophil Dermatosis

Initial Therapy

1. Oral prednisone 40–60 mg/day will result in a dramatic clinical response in 24–48 hours.
2. Continue prednisone at the initial dose until lesions have completely or almost completely resolved.

Subsequent Therapy

1. After response, reduce prednisone by 10-mg increments each week over the next 4–6 weeks to the dose necessary to control the disorder. Most patients will be completely weaned from steroids in 6–8 weeks.
2. Relapse may require reinstitution of steroids and another attempt at tapering medication to the control dose.
3. Patients requiring long-term systemic steroids are most safely treated with q.o.d. therapy.

Alternative Therapy

There are no truly effective alternative treatments. Aspirin, indomethacin, colchicine, and potassium iodide have, however, been reported to be useful in isolated situations.

Pitfalls

1. Complications of therapy are those of chronic systemic steroid use as outlined in Appendix 5.
2. Sweet syndrome may be associated with acute myelogenous leukemia, and may present during a leukemic or preleukemic state. These patients are frequently anemic.

BW

168

Syphilis

Lues

The treatment of syphilis is based on the duration of infection and the organ systems involved. Five groups can be distinguished: primary, secondary, or early syphilis of less than 1 year's duration; infection of indeterminate length, or more than 1 year's duration;

neurosyphilis; congenital syphilis; and syphilis infection in association with HIV infection. In all cases of syphilis it is important to examine for and treat other STDs, and to trace and treat all contacts. Syphilis cases should be reported to the local health department. Infected individuals may resume sexual activity after skin lesions, if present, are healed, or after therapy is complete.

Initial Therapy

PRIMARY, SECONDARY, OR EARLY SYPHILIS

1. Intramuscular benzathine penicillin G 2.4×10^6 U as a single dose. Some experts feel a second 2.4×10^6-U dose 1 week later leads to enhanced clinical and serologic cures.
2. Penicillin-allergic patients: oral tetracycline HCl 500 mg q.i.d. for 15 days.
3. For penicillin-allergic pregnant patients only: oral erythromycin 500 mg q.i.d. for 15 days. Erythromycin may not adequately treat the fetus. Give additional penicillin therapy as for congenital syphilis (see below) to the baby at birth.

INFECTION OF INDETERMINATE LENGTH, OR MORE THAN 1 YEAR'S DURATION

1. Intramuscular benzathine penicillin G 2.4×10^6 U/week for 3 successive weeks.
2. Penicillin-allergic patients: oral tetracycline HCl 500 mg q.i.d. for 30 days.
3. For penicillin-allergic pregnant patients only: oral erythromycin 500 mg q.i.d. for 30 days.

NEUROSYPHILIS

Neurosyphilis may occur at any time during syphilitic infection. Diagnosis requires a reactive CSF with increased cell count, increased protein content, and a positive CSF VDRL. The serum FTA-ABS or MHA-TP is positive in all cases. Neurologically normal patients with early syphilis do not require CSF examination. CSF examination is required during and after treatments as an index of cure.

Preferred Therapy

Intravenous aqueous penicillin G 4×10^6 U q.4h. for 14 days.

Alternative Therapy

Intramuscular procaine penicillin G 2.4×10^6 U/day with oral probenecid 500 mg q.i.d. for 14 days.

3. For penicillin-allergic patients: Oral tetracycline HCl 500 mg q.i.d. for 30 days.
4. For penicillin-allergic pregnant patients: Oral erythromycin 500 mg q.i.d. for 30 days.

CONGENITAL SYPHILIS

Infected infants may be asymptomatic at birth and have negative serologic studies. The initial evaluation requires:

1. A physical examination.
2. Maternal history to include serologic status, treatment, and response to treatment. Adequate treatment of the mother before delivery, except with erythromycin, treats the infant, although if treatment is delayed until late in gestation, stigmata may still appear.
3. CSF examination for cells, protein, and VDRL.
4. Radiographs of the long bones.
5. Examination of any lesions for spirochetes by darkfield (e.g., snuffles) or histologic special stains. A positive CSF VDRL in the asymptomatic infant requires treatment for possible CNS involvement (regimen b, below).
   a. Infants with normal CSF: Intramuscular benzathine penicillin G 50,000 U/kg in a single dose.
   b. Infants with abnormal CSF and those in whom CNS involvement cannot be ruled out: Intramuscular aqueous procaine penicillin G 50,000 U/kg/day for 10 days.
   c. For older children the dosage of penicillin is as noted above, but should not exceed that recommended for adults with syphilis of more than 1 year's duration.

SYPHILIS IN THE HIV-INFECTED INDIVIDUAL

HIV infection may alter the natural history of syphilis in two ways: A negative VDRL or RPR can occur with active secondary syphilis; and early CNS relapse after apparently adequate therapy has been observed on multiple occasions.

Initial Therapy

1. The current CDC guidelines recommend no change in therapy for early syphilis in the HIV-infected individual (see above). It may be prudent to treat all HIV-infected individuals with early syphilis with three consecutive, weekly, intramuscular injections of benzathine penicillin 2.4×10^6 U. Therapeutic failure with oral erythromycin has been reported.
2. A CSF examination should precede and guide treatment of HIV-infected individuals with latent syphilis or syphilis present for 1 year or more, or of unknown duration. If CSF examination is not possible, treat for presumed neurosyphilis.
3. Do not use benzathine penicillin to treat neurosyphilis in the HIV-infected individual. See treatment regimen c, above.
4. HIV-positive persons with CNS findings should be evaluated for possible neurosyphilis.
5. Notify state epidemiologists of any HIV-infected patient with neurosyphilis or seronegative-documented secondary syphilis.

Alternative Therapy

Use only the standard regimens noted above. Efficacy of other regimens is not established.

Subsequent Therapy

1. All patients require repeat serum VDRL determinations: for those with early syphilis and congenital syphilis, at 3, 6, and 12 months; for those with syphilis of more than 1 year's duration at 12 and 24 months; for pregnant patients, monthly until delivery; for HIV-infected individuals at 1, 2, and 3 months, and at 3-month intervals until a two-dilution or greater decrease in VDRL titer occurs. Thereafter every 6 months until seronegative.
2. For all patients with neurosyphilis, and infants with possible neurosyphilis, in addition, a CSF examination must be repeated 6 months following treatment. Adequate therapy is determined by a normal CSF cell count and a falling protein content. The VDRL may not return to negative. CSF examination in documented neurosyphilis (with abnormal CSF findings) is continued at 6-month intervals for 2 years. A normal CSF at 1 year is evidence of cure.

Pitfalls

1. Compliance with long courses of oral antibiotics is a concern. Parenteral treatment is preferred. If oral therapy is given, compliance must be stressed, and careful follow-up is essential to document cure.

2. Tetracycline is contraindicated in pregnancy and in children under 8 years of age.
3. A Jarisch-Herxheimer reaction may occur in the first 24 hours after treating any patient. Patients should be warned before therapy. The treatment is bed rest and aspirin. Do *not* discontinue therapy.

TB

169

Systemic Lupus Erythematosus

In patients with systemic lupus erythematosus (SLE), the cutaneous lesions usually respond to therapy of the systemic process.

Initial Therapy

1. Prednisone 60 mg/day in divided t.i.d. or q.i.d. doses is usually adequate to control moderate-to-severe disease accompanied by involvement of one or more internal organs. Taper the dose as clinical and laboratory parameters normalize to the lowest possible dose (a typical maintenance dose is 7.5 mg b.i.d.). Eventually make an attempt to reduce this dose as well, because some patients can be completely withdrawn from steroids. *Note:* q.o.d. regimens are usually not effective in achieving disease control.
2. The cutaneous manifestations of SLE often respond to applications of superpotent topical steroids (see Appendix 1).
3. For patients with disfiguring dermatologic abnormalities, give antimalarials in addition to corticosteroids (see Ch. 48, Discoid Lupus Erythematosus).
4. *Lupus panniculitis* is a localized form of SLE or an extension of DLE. When panniculitis is the primary or sole manifestation of SLE, therapy with hydroxychloroquine (Plaquenil) 200 mg/day alone often suffices to control disease.
5. Perform a work-up on all patients suspected of having SLE for both the presence of antinuclear antibodies and the Ro antibody system. Serologic tests should include an ANA and a screen for the presence of antibodies against native DNA, ENA Ro (SSA), and La (SSB). In addition, serum complement levels should be obtained (CH50, C3, C4); all patients with low complement levels should be evaluated for possible glomerulonephritis.

Alternative Therapy

1. Corticosteroid "pulse-therapy" (see Ch. 149) may be helpful in patients whose disease is not controlled with prednisone doses of 80 mg/day or less.
2. Cyclophosphamide, with oral corticosteroids (see dosages above), is especially useful for patients with vasculitis of medium-to-large vessels.
3. Plasmaphoresis, if combined with corticosteroid and/or immunosuppressive therapy (cylophosphamide 1–2 mg/kg/day or azathioprine 50–150 mg/day), may be useful in refractory cases.

Subsequent Therapy

1. SLE patients with lupus profundus, recalcitrant discoid lesions, or alopecia may need additional intralesional therapy (triaminolone acetonide, 2.5 mg/cc, administered using a 30-gauge needle).
2. Sunscreens, with protection against both UVB and UVA, and with a protective rating of 15 or greater, should be employed daily.
3. Aspirin in anti-inflammatory doses or other NSAIDs may be used if arthritis flares as corticosteroids are tapered.

Ancillary Therapy

1. Adequate rest during active disease is important.
2. Women should avoid pregnancy unless disease is in remission and steroid (prednisone) dose is less than 15 mg/day. All other drugs also should be stopped prior to pregnancy. When patients with SLE become pregnant (and for 6 weeks postpartum), laboratory parameters of disease activity must be monitored frequently and intravenous corticosteroids should be administered during labor.
3. Patients with SLE should be monitored for infections, and antibiotic prophylaxis is indicated in patients on systemic corticosteroids during dental procedures.

Pitfalls

1. Either vitiligo-like depigmentation or hyperpigmentation can remain at sites of previously active disease sites.
2. Annular forms of subacute lupus can be confused with erythema multiforme, figurate erythemas, granuloma annulare, or sarcoidosis.
3. Several, rare, inherited, early-component complement disorders are associated with some clinical features of SLE or subacute lupus. Also, maternal carriers of chronic granulomatous disease of childhood may display cutaneous features of SLE.

4. A number of associated skin conditions, such as Raynaud syndrome, digital infarcts, urticaria, alopecia, sclerodactyly, and calcinosis cutis can occur in SLE.
5. SLE can enter a fulminant phase after acute or excessive exposure to sunlight.
6. The pitfalls of corticosteroid therapy are discussed in Appendices 3, 4, and 5.
7. The pitfalls of antimalarials are discussed in Chapter 48.
8. The pitfalls of immunosuppressive therapy are discussed in Appendix 7. In addition to hemorrhagic cystitis, cyclophosphamide may be associated with an increased incidence of sarcoma and leukemia.

PE

170

Tattoos

All therapies for the removal of tattoos are surgical.

Initial Therapy

Simple excision in one or multiple stages (3–12 months apart) gives a predictable result. Since most tattoos are on the extremities, the scars may spread. Prior placement of tissue expanders may give adequate tissue for reduced-tension closure.

Alternative Therapy

1. *Superficial* dermabrasion *to the papillary dermis,* followed by the application of a styptic and gentian violet. An eschar forms, often with the tattoo pigment in it, reproducing the figure of the tatoo. This superficial abrasion may be repeated on several occasions to remove additional pigment.
2. A superficial salabrasion may be performed to remove the epidermis and part of the papillary dermis. This gives similar results to dermabrasion.
3. Currently laser removal of tattoos does not predictably produce superior cosmetic results to the procedures outlined above.

4. For very large tattoos a dermatome may be used to shave off a split thickness of skin, which is allowed to heal with an eschar as above.

Pitfalls

1. Patients should be counselled that all methods except complete excision may leave residual pigment. Abrasion procedures tend to work best on professional tattoos with a more even depth of pigment.
2. Hypertrophic scarring, keloid formation, and hypopigmentation may follow any form of tattoo removal, and patients should be so counselled.
3. Careful selection of patients prior to surgery (including perhaps a psychiatric evaluation) may avoid postsurgical patient dissatisfaction. Pre- and postoperative photographs and documented fully informed consent are essential.

TB

171

Thrush

Oral Candidiasis

Thrush occurs in infants, diabetics, immunosuppressed persons, and following oral antibiotic or steroid therapy.

Initial Therapy

1. For infants, oral nystatin suspension (100,000 U/ml) 2 ml q.i.d. for 1 week.
2. For others, Nystatin suspension (100,000 u/ml) 5 ml (1 tsp) swish and swallow q.i.d. for 1–2 weeks.

Alternative Therapy

1. For adults, clotrimazole troches (dissolved in the mouth) 2–5×/day.
2. For refractory cases, ketaconazole tables 200 mg b.i.d. for 1–2 weeks.

Pitfalls

1. In the edentulous, dentures may be a reservoir for candidiasis and need to be cleaned daily and coated with nystatin ointment for 1 week.
2. Evaluate for immunosuppression if other associated conditions are not present.
3. Clotrimazole troches and oral ketaconazole may cause elevated LFT levels.

TB

172

Tinea Capitis

Tinea capitis is much more common in children than adults. Two forms are recognized, a noninflammatory and an inflammatory type.

BLACK-DOT (NONINFLAMMATORY TINEA CAPITIS)

Initial Therapy

1. Griseofulvin, ultramicromized (e.g., Gris-Peg) 10–15 mg/kg/day is the treatment of choice. For children unable to swallow capsules, the pills are crushed and put in food. Therapy is given in a b.i.d. regimen with meals, and continued for at least 6 weeks, or until cultures are negative.
2. Selenium sulfide 2% shampoo (Selsun) q.d. or q.o.d.

Alternative Therapy

1. Ketoconazole (Nizoral) 200 mg/day for adults (or 3.3 mg/kg/day for children) is as effective as griseofulvin, but should be reserved for adult cases of tinea capitis.

Ancillary Therapy

1. Examine, culture, and treat any family members who are infected.

2. Brushes, combs, and hats should be cleaned, and family members should be instructed not to share these items.

KERION (INFLAMMATORY TINEA CAPITIS)

Initial Therapy

1. Antifungal therapy with griseofulvin or ketoconazole, as above.
2. If substantial areas of the scalp are involved, systemic corticosteroids (prednisone 1–2 mg/kg/day), in a single dose, should be given for 1 week or until inflammation subsides. Then, taper over 1–2 weeks.

Ancillary Therapy

1. Bacterial secondary infection is uncommon. Do not use antibiotics unless the patient has both tenderness and fever, as well as positive cultures of purulent material.
2. Compresses with Domeboro (diluted 1:40) should be used if substantial oozing and crusts are present.
3. Selenium sulfide 2% (Selsun) shampoo, as described above.
4. Family members should be examined for possible infection, and if infected, treated as above.
5. Brushes, combs, and hats should be cleaned and not shared among family members.

PITFALLS

For pitfalls of systemic griseofulvin and ketoconazole therapy, see Chapters 32 and 175, respectively.

PE

173

Tinea Corporis and Tinea Cruris

Tinea corporis and cruris can occur alone or in conjunction with other dermatophyte infections (e.g., tinea pedis).

Initial Therapy

1. Topical antifungals: Newer imidazole and related agents (see Appendix 2), are more effective than tolnaftate (Tinactin) or undecenylate (Desenex) preparations. Although solutions or lotions usually are preferable to creams because of their superior ability to access fissures and scaling areas, unfortunately, some of the most effective topical agents currently are available only in cream formulations. When a cream formulation is appropriate, miconazole (Micatin) is preferred initially because of its relatively low cost and availability without a prescription. The antifungal agent should be applied b.i.d., once immediately after bathing, and one additional time approximately 12 hours later.

2. Tinea corporis and cruris infections may be resistant to topical medications alone, suggesting a degree of impaired host immunity against the agent in their pathogenesis. Hence, a 3–6-week course of either griseofulvin (500 mg micronized or 250 mg ultramicronized b.i.d. (Grispeg)) or ketoconazole (Nizoral) 200–400 mg/day may be necessary to achieve clearing.

Ancillary Therapy

Dermatophytes thrive in a humid, warm environment. Hence, patients should be encouraged to apply a drying powder (e.g., Zeasorb) q.d. or b.i.d. to intertriginous areas if infected, and to allow as much air to reach affected sites as possible.

Subsequent Therapy

1. Topical antifungals always should be used in conjunction with systemic antifungal therapy to allow early discontinuation of systemic antifungals.
2. Topical and ancillary measures may need to be continued indefinitely to achieve total clearing and/or to prevent recurrences.

3. Some tinea corporis infections can be obtained from animals; hence, household animals should be examined for skin infections, and treated appropriately.

Pitfalls

1. Tinea corporis clinically can resemble nummular eczema, pityriasis rosea, or secondary syphilis. Tinea cruris can resemble candidiasis, erythrasma, seborrheic dermatitis, lichen simplex chronicus (neurodermatitis), and rarely Hailey-Hailey disease or localized forms of histiocytosis X. A positive KOH examination or culture is recommended before initiating systemic antifungal therapy.
2. Both griseofulvin and ketoconazole can cause serious side effects, toxicity, and important drug interactions (see Chs. 32 and 175, Coccidiomycosis and Tinea Pedis respectively). The treating physician needs to be acquainted with these before prescribing either of these agents.

PE

174

Tinea Manuum

Tinea manuum usually presents as part of the two foot-one hand syndrome, with coexistent tinea pedis (see Ch. 175, Tinea Pedis).

Initial Therapy

1. Topical antifungals: Imidazole agents (see Appendix 2) are more effective than tolnaftate (Tinactin) or undecenylate preparations (e.g., Desenex). Although solutions or lotions usually are preferable to creams because of their superior ability to access fissures and scaling areas, unfortunately, some of the most effective topical agents currently are available only in cream formulations. When a cream formulation is appropriate, miconazole (Micatin) is preferred because of its relatively low cost and availability without a prescription. The antifungal agent should be applied b.i.d.,

once immediately after bathing, and one additional time approximately 12 hours later.

2. Tinea manuum is notoriously resistant to topical antifungals alone, suggesting a degree of impaired host immunity in its pathogenesis. Hence, a 6–12 week course of either griseofulvin 500 mg micronized or 250 mg ultramicronized (Grispeg) b.i.d. or ketoconazole (Nizoral) 200 mg/day may be necessary to achieve clearing.

Subsequent Therapy

Systemic therapy should be discontinued after clearing has occurred, but topical antifungal therapy needs to be continued indefinitely or relapses are likely.

Pitfalls

1. Tinea manuum tends to recur, and repeated courses of therapy may be needed.
2. Both griseofulvin and ketoconazole can cause serious side effects, toxicity, and serious drug interactions (see Chs. 175 and 31). The treating physician needs to be acquainted with these before prescribing either of these agents.

PE

175

Tinea Pedis

This chapter provides therapeutic guidelines for the therapy of tinea pedis (see Chs. 127–174 and 176 and 177 for therapy for tinea capitis, tinea corporis, tinea manuum, tinea versicolor, and tinea unguium (onychomycosis)). *Note:* Tinea pedis is an important potential portal of entry for bacterial pathogens, and as a result, cellulitis, lymphangitis, and even sepsis can result, particularly in elderly patients with pre-existing lymphedema.

Initial Therapy

Topical antifungals: Imidazole agents are more effective than tolnaftate (Tinactin) or undecenylate preparations (e.g., Desenex). Although solutions or lotions usually are preferable to creams because of their superior ability to access fissures and scaling areas, unfortuntely, some of the more effective topical agents are available currently only in cream formulations. Where a cream formulation is appropriate, miconazole (Micatin) is preferred because of its relatively low cost and availability without a prescription. The antifungal agent should be applied b.i.d., once immediately after bathing, and one additional time approximately 12 hours later.

Alternative Therapy

Many tinea infections are resistant to topical medications alone, suggesting a degree of impaired host resistance in their pathogenesis. Hence, supplement topical therapy with a 3–6-week course of either griseofulvin 500 mg micronized or 250 mg ultramicronized (Grispeg) b.i.d. or ketoconazole (Nizoral) 200 mg/day in recurrent cases and in cases resistant to topical therapy alone.

Ancillary Therapy

Dermatophytes thrive in a humid, warm environment. Therefore, encourage patients to apply a drying powder (e.g., Zeasorb) q.d. or b.i.d. to affected areas when appropriate (for tinea cruris or tinea pedis), and to allow as much air to reach affected sites as possible (i.e., with tinea pedis: remove shoes as soon as arriving home; with tinea cruris: wear boxer shorts, loose-fitting trousers, etc.).

Subsequent Therapy

1. Use all of the topical measures described under Initial Therapy in conjunction with systemic therapy to allow discontinuation of oral antifungals after a response occurs.
2. Topical and preventive measures may need to be continued indefinitely to achieve total clearing and/or to prevent recurrences.
3. Some tinea infections can be obtained from household animals; hence, household animals should be examined for skin infections and treated appropriately.

Pitfalls

1. Superficial fungal infections (except for tinea corporis) tend to recur, and repeated courses of therapy may be needed. The ancillary, preventive measures described above may decrease the frequency and/or severity of recurrences.
2. As noted above, tinea pedis is an important "portal of entry" for potentially devastating bacterial infections, particularly in the elderly. Hence, aggressive therapy is indicated; these are not trivial infections!
3. Both griseofulvin and ketoconazole can cause serious side effects, toxicity, and important drug interactions (See Chapters 175 and 31, respectively, for discussion). The treating physician needs to be acquainted with these before prescribing either of these agents.

PE

176

Tinea Unguium

Onychomycosis

It is not necessary or appropriate to treat most cases of tinea ungium of the toenail, which in any case, is extremely difficult to eradicate. Treatment of fingernails has a far greater likelihood of success.

Initial Therapy

1. Because of the possible toxicity from long-term therapy with systemic antifungal antibiotics, it is necessary to obtain a positive KOH preparation or culture prior to initiating therapy.
2. Griseofulvin 500 mg b.i.d. of an ultramicronized preparation is taken as a single daily dose with meals.
3. Attempt chemical debridement of toenail lesions by application of a thick layer of 40% urea in petrolatum or aquaphor cream to the affected nail(s). The nail is kept occluded, while the surrounding skin is protected with adhesive tape. After 1 week the diseased nail(s) is(are) avulsed. A second

application of the urea cream may be needed for an additional week to achieve complete chemical debridement.

4. After the nail has been avulsed, apply a topical imidazole solution (see Appendix 2) to the nail bed b.i.d.

Alternate Therapy

1. Ketoconazole 200 mg q.d. or b.i.d. is as effective as griseofulvin, and may be effective in cases that do not respond to griseofulvin.
2. Carbon dioxide laser can be used for debridement of diseased nails, but must be supplemented with oral and topical antifungal agents.

Ancillary Therapy

1. Thymol 5% in absolute ethyl alcohol, applied q.d. or b.i.d., may provide additional antifungal activity.
2. For tinea unguium of the toenails, an important goal of therapy is to restrict infection to the involved nail(s). A drying, antifungal powder (e.g., Desenex or Tinactin), should be added to the stockings daily. In addition, patients should remove shoes whenever possible to maximize aeration.

PE

177

Tinea Versicolor

Pityrosporum Folliculitis

TINEA VERSICOLOR

Initial Therapy

1. Selenium sulfide shampoo is the most economical therapy and many treatment schedules are effective. Have the patient apply the shampoo to wet skin from the ear lobes to the knees and wrists with a scrub brush or pad (e.g., Buf Puf) at bedtime to loosen hyphae, let it dry, and sleep with it on

overnight. In the morning the shampoo is showered off and the scalp (and beard) are shampooed for 5 minutes with the selenium sulfide shampoo. Shampoos containing zinc pyrithione or sulfur and salicylic acid are probably equally effective.

2. Oral ketaconazole is very effective and may be used alone or in addition to the above treatment. Several treatment schedules are effective. Give the patient 2–4 tablets (400–800 mg) to be taken at one time. The patient exercises 20–30 minutes after taking the tablets to the point of sweating. The sweat is allowed to dry on the skin and washed off after at least several hours.

3. Launder all underclothing, sheets, and towels.

4. Evaluate other family members for infection. It may be asymptomatic.

Alternative Therapy

1. Shampoos containing selenium sulfide, zinc pyrithione, or sulfur and salicylic acid may be applied for 10–20 minutes/day followed by a shampooing for 2 weeks.

2. Oral ketaconazole 200 mg q.h.s. for 2 weeks is very effective.

3. Benzoyl peroxide 5%–10% q.d. for 1 month may be used.

4. Sodium thiosulfate 25%–30% solution b.i.d. for 4–6 weeks.

Subsequent Therapy

1. Although many treatment regimens clear the condition, reappearance of the infection is extremely common especially during the warm seasons or in tropical climates. For this reason all patients are instructed on prophylactic measures, which include:

   a. Oral ketoconazole 200 mg for 3 consecutive days every month, or

   b. Once-monthly application of the above-mentioned shampoos overnight or for 30 minutes before showering.

   These are used all year around by those who regularly exercise and during the warm months only by others.

2. Postinfection hypo- or hyperpigmentation is common. Inform patients that this will resolve over several months after adequate treatment.

Pitfalls

1. Oral ketaconazole is rarely associated with hepatotoxicity. It should not be routinely used in those with known liver disease. LFTs should be monitored in patients using it longer than 2–4 weeks. Men should be informed of the potential of reversible decreased libido.

2. Many patients referred to dermatologists for resistant tinea versicolor (TV) have only persistent hypopigmentation. This is treated with watchful waiting, support, and suppression of recurrences.

PITYROSPORUM FOLLICULITIS

Occasionally the organism causing TV will cause a folliculitis without the typical dermatitis of TV. Topicals are not uniformly effective.

Initial Therapy

1. Oral ketaconazole 200–400 mg/day for 2–3 weeks.
2. Topical benzoyl peroxide 5%–10% gel q.h.s. may be adjunctively beneficial.

Pitfalls

Suspect pityrosporum folliculitis in culture-negative acute or chronic folliculitis and do a biopsy to confirm it.

TB

178

Toxic Epidermal Necrolysis

Toxic epidermal necrolysis (TEN) is almost always drug induced, although other factors can contribute to its pathogenesis. TEN can be differentiated from generalized staphylococcal scalded skin syndrome by the presence of full-thickness epidermal necrosis on histology or cytology (Tzanck smear). Management of TEN is best accomplished in a burn unit, where therapy appropriate for an extensive 100% second-degree burn can be provided.

Initial Therapy

1. Placement in an in-patient unit, specialized in the management of burn victims.

2. Monitoring and replacement of fluid, electrolytes, and colloids, based upon assessment of central venous pressure, urine output, blood pressure, and weight.

3. Conservative debridement of loosely attached, nonviable, necrolytic, epidermolytic sheets. Leave intact bullae in place, as they provide an optimal barrier.

4. Application of pigskin xenografts or homologous human skin grafts (if available) to denuded areas.

5. Frequent monitoring for secondary infection and/or possible sepsis (in the presence of generalized necrolysis normal thermoregulatory mechanisms may be absent; therefore, core temperature may not reflect presence of infection). Obtain repeated cultures of blood, skin, and urine, and initiate parenteral antibiotic therapy empirically with broad-spectrum coverage for both gram-positive and negative pathogens at earliest signs of infection.

Subsequent Therapy

1. Stop the most likely offending drugs (sulfonamides, anticonvulsives, analgesics, allopurinol, and penicillins, in order of likelihood).

2. Give consideration to early institution of plasmapheresis, as recent uncontrolled studies seem to indicate improved mortality statistics with this therapeutic modality.

Ancillary Measures

1. Mucosal involvement can be severe; therefore, oral cleansing and antisepsis are critical. Ophthalmic sequelae, however, do not seem to be as severe as in Stevens-Johnson syndrome. *Note:* Topical sulfonamide eyedrops are to be avoided in patients with possible sulfonamide-induced TEN.

2. Scarring sequelae (anonychia, milia, scarring) can be severe and disfiguring. Whether a large bolus of systemic steroids (e.g., methylprednisolone 1 g in 150 ml of 5% dextrose in water, infused over 1 hour) will reduce late sequelae—or mortality for that matter–is still not known.

Pitfalls

1. Deaths in TEN patients are primarily due to sepsis, often as a consequence of prior high-dose systemic steroid therapy. Hence, *on-going steroid therapy, which has never proven to be of benefit, is contraindicated.* However, an initial bolus of steroids should not carry this risk (see above), and might reduce sequelae, as well as possibly improve overall survival rate.

2. The other two major causes of mortality are upper GI bleeding (Curling's

ulcers, also usually attributable to the use of steroids), and renal failure, secondary to hypovolemia and inadequate attention to fluid and electrolytic status.
3. Some patients with TEN experience recurrent attacks, usually when the offending drug is readministered. Thus, all TEN patients should carry warning cards and wear Medic-Alert bracelets.

PE

179

Transient Acantholytic Dermatosis

Grover's Disease

Lesions of transient acantholytic dermatosis (TAD) often are not "transient," and may persist for years. Some cases are clearly exacerbated by heat or sunlight, and pruritus may be severe.

Initial Therapy

1. A high-potency or superpotent steroid cream, applied b.i.d., is effective in most patients, and may suffice for patients with limited numbers of lesions.
2. For patients with extensive disease, isotretinoin 40 mg/day is given for 2 weeks or until improvement occurs (not to exceed 12 weeks). If improvement occurs by 2 weeks, begin to taper to 10 mg/day over the next month, then maintain at this dose for a total of 12 weeks of therapy.

Alternative Therapy

1. Oral vitamin A 50,000 U t.i.d. for 2 weeks, followed by reduction to 50,000 U q.d. for a total of 12 weeks.
2. Methotrexate (25–50 mg/week) in a single dose or a divided-dose regimen is effective in some refractory cases.

3. Photochemotherapy (PUVA) is effective in some cases; an initial brief exacerbation may occur, however, before clearing.
4. Systemic steroids can provide temporary relief, but relapses generally occur.

Ancillary Therapy

1. An emollient lotion, containing menthol, phenol, and camphor (e.g., Sarna), may provide temporary relief.
2. Antihistamines (e.g., doxepin 25 mg q.h.s., oral chlorpheniramine 4–8 mg t.i.d., or terphenadine (Seldane) 60 mg b.i.d. or t.i.d.) (the last is particularly useful when soporific effects need to be avoided).
3. Avoidance of excess sunlight and use of broad-spectrum sunscreens (SPF of 15 or greater) may prevent exacerbations.

Pitfalls

1. TAD, despite its name, may not be transient, and may persist for years.
2. The potential side effects of systemic retinoids, methotrexate, and topical and systemic steroids are discussed in Appendices 3, 5, 6, 7.

PE

180

Uremic Pruritus

Uremic pruritus is encountered in patients with severe renal failure. Although hemodialysis may offer some relief, uremic pruritus is frequent during chronic dialysis. The goal of therapy is relief of pruritus.

Initial Therapy

1. Treat dry skin with hydration and emollients.
   a. Tub-soak for 15–20 minutes b.i.d. in comfortably warm water without soap.
   b. Pat dry, and immediately apply an emollient (e.g., Eucerin).

2. An antihistamine (e.g., hydroxyzine (Atarax) 25 mg b.i.d. or t.i.d.) may be useful.

Alternative Therapy

If symptoms are not relieved by hydration and bland emollients within 2–3 weeks, the following measures are reasonable alternatives.

1. Apply a medium-potency topical steroid in an ointment b.i.d. Improvement will be noted within 7–14 days. If the patient responds, attempt to replace the topical steroids with emollient and hydration.
2. UVB irradiation benefits many patients.
    a. Begin UVB exposure at 75% of the estimated minimal erythema dose (MED) (see Ch. 147, Psoriasis).
    b. Treat 3x/week, gradually increasing UVB exposure; pruritus will be relieved within 6–8 treatments.
    c. Remissions may last months to years; relapses in patients who have experienced previous UVB-mediated remissions will often respond to additional courses of UVB therapy.
3. Cholestyramine (Questran) 4 g (1 packet) t.i.d. before meals may provide relief.

Other Therapy

Subtotal parathyroidectomy may relieve pruritus if the symptoms are due to secondary hyperparathyroidism.

BW

181

Urticaria

Acute Urticaria • Chronic Urticaria • Cold Urticaria • Cholinergic Urticaria • Pressure Urticaria • Hives

Urticaria ("hives") may be acute or chronic, or may result from physical stimuli. Although initial treatment of these entities is similar, subsequent therapeutic alternatives differ significantly as outlined below.

ACUTE URTICARIA

Acute urticaria results from a variety of causes including drug reactions, food allergy, systemic disorders, and undetermined causes, and may be a component of anaphylactic reaction. Following discontinuation of the inciting agent, the majority of acute reactions resolve within days to weeks. Therefore, therapy is symptomatic and attempts to suppress symptoms until urticaria abates.

Initial Therapy

1. Treat with an H_1 antagonist antihistamine. Hydroxyzine (Atarax) 25 mg t.i.d. or q.i.d. will usually suppress pruritus and all or the majority of cutaneous lesions.
2. If urticaria is suppressed, treat the patient continually in order to maintain control of the process.

Subsequent Therapy

1. If urticaria is not suppressed satisfactorily, increase hydroxyzine every 3–4 days to a maximum of 200 mg/day.
2. After 2–3 weeks of satisfactory suppression of urticaria, discontinue antihistamines. If urticaria recurs, restart antihistamines and attempt to wean patient from medication after an additional 3 weeks.

Alternative Therapy

Occasionally the severity of urticarial lesions will require more aggressive therapy, or patients will not be adequately controlled by the H_1 receptor antagonist alone.

1. Treat with a combination of hydroxyzine 25–50 mg q.i.d. and cyproheptadine (Periactin) 4 mg q.i.d.
2. Treat with other H_1 receptor antagonists. Diphenhydramine (Benadryl) 25–50 mg q.i.d. or tripelennamine (Pyribenzamine) 25–50 mg t.i.d. are excellent choices. Astemazole (Hismanal) 10–20 mg/day or terfenadine (Seldane) 60–120 mg b.i.d. are nonsedating H_1 antagonists that may be useful.
3. In the event of failure of H_1 antagonists, oral doxepin (Sinequan) may be useful. Begin therapy with 25 mg b.i.d. and increase the dose every 4–5 days to a maximum of 50 mg t.i.d. Because doxepin can prolong the PR interval and worsen conduction defects, obtain an ECG prior to therapy with doxepin.
4. In unusually severe, unresponsive cases, prednisone 60 mg/day in a single dose or divided dose may be necessary to control urticaria. As soon as urtication is controlled, taper steroids over a 7–14-day period.

Pitfalls

1. If urticaria is not suppressed by initial doses of an H_1 antihistamine, increase the dose to the limit of side effects tolerated by the patient. The majority of acute urticarial reactions will not require use of epinephrine or systemic steroids.
2. Acute urticaria may be a manifestation of systemic anaphylaxis. In such situations, treat the patient rapidly for this potentially fatal disorder.
3. Other systemic disorders may present as acute urticaria. Look for immune-complex diseases and the initial phase of viral hepatitis in patients with symptoms not clearly explained by urticaria.
4. Drowsiness is a frequent complication of antihistamine therapy, but often resolves with continuation of therapy.
5. Look for drugs that cause or exacerbate urticaria (including such commonly used agents as salicylates and NSAIDS).

CHRONIC URTICARIA

This disorder is defined as urticaria lasting longer than 6 weeks; the cause is often not found. The goal of therapy is to provide relief of symptoms.

Initial Therapy

Treat with an H_1 antihistamine receptor antagonist. Because hydroxyzine (Atarax) is an effective, inexpensive antihistamine, begin with 25–50 mg t.i.d. or q.i.d., depending on the severity of urticaria and the patient's tolerance of somnolent side effects. Diphenhydramine (Benadryl) 25–50 mg q.i.d., tripelennamine (Pyribenzamine) 25–50 mg t.i.d., chlorpheniramine (Chlor-Trimeton) 8–12 mg/day, and the nonsedating agents terfenadine (Seldane) 60–120 mg b.i.d., and astemazole 10–20 mg q.d. offer appropriate initial choices. Emphasize that the antihistamine be taken as directed rather than on a p.r.n. basis, and that the goal of treatment is suppression of itching rather than the complete suppression of hives.

Subsequent Therapy

1. If symptoms are suppressed and no urticaria is present, continue antihistamine treatment at the lowest possible regular dose for 4–6 weeks, then discontinue antihistamines.
2. If urticaria recurs, treat for an additional 6–8 weeks and attempt to discontinue medication. This cycle may be repeated as often as needed.

Alternative Therapy

An H_1 antagonist alone may not be adequate. The following alternatives are reasonable.

1. Add cyproheptadine (Periactin) 4 mg q.i.d. to a maximum of 32 mg/day.
2. Add an H_2 receptor antagonist. Cimetidine (Tagamet) 300 mg q.i.d. or ranitidine (Zantac) 150–300 mg b.i.d. may be of value.
3. Doxepin (Sinequan), a tricyclic antidepressent, is an effective antihistamine. Treat initially with 25 mg b.i.d. if tolerated and gradually increase to a maximum of 50 mg t.i.d. Because this agent lengthens the PR interval, obtain an initial ECG and recheck in older individuals as the dose is raised.
4. If antihistamines alone do not control urticarial symptoms, prednisone 40 mg q.a.m. for 3 days is reasonable therapy. After 3 days, reduce dose by 5 mg/day until 25 mg/day is reached. Then reduce dose by 5 mg q.o.d. until 25 mg q.o.d. is reached. Next, decrease prednisone to the lowest dose that controls symptoms and attempt to discontinue therapy every 2–3 months.
5. Elimination diets and skin testing may be done in recalcitrant cases and are best carried out under the supervision of an allergist.

Pitfalls

1. Look for drugs that aggravate or cause urticaria. Salicylates are the best known.
2. Doxepin lengthens the PR interval, and can cause sudden death in patients with a history of cardiac arrhythmias. Obtain an ECG prior to institution of this drug, and recheck as the dose is increased.
3. Cyproheptadine is a known appetite stimulant. This can be troublesome, particularly in patients on concomitant steroids.
4. Chronic urticaria may be caused by vasculitis. True urticarial lesions last less than 24 hours. Urticaria lasting more than 24 hours requires a biopsy to rule out vasculitis.

COLD URTICARIA

Initial Therapy

The initial treatment of choice is cyproheptadine (Periactin). Begin with 4 mg q.i.d. and increase to a maximum total dose of 32 mg/day. Most patients will benefit from this therapy.

Alternative Therapy

In the event of incomplete or unsatisfactory response to cyproheptadine, try the following alternatives.

1. Add doxepin 25–50 mg q.h.s.
2. Although not of frequent benefit, try cimetidine (Tagamet) 300 mg b.i.d. to q.i.d.

CHOLINERGIC URTICARIA

The drug of choice is oral hydroxyzine (Atarax) 25–100 mg q.i.d. For unexplained reasons, other antihistamines are far less useful. In the event of failure of response, alternatives are those described for treatment of chronic urticaria.

PRESSURE URTICARIA/ANGIOEDEMA

While antihistamines are usually tried initially, they usually do not work. This disorder responds to systemic steroids, and the decision to use these agents depends on the severity of the disorder, the degree of disability, and the amount of steroids required for satisfactory control.

If steroid therapy is elected, begin with prednisone 0.5–1.0 mg/kg/day for 7–10 days. Decrease dose to 20 mg q.o.d. If control is maintained, decrease prednisone by 2.5 mg/week until the minimum amount of prednisone is reached. Some patients may be controlled by as little as 7.5 mg q.o.d., while others may require 35–40 mg q.o.d. Rare individuals in whom side effects of the drug are outweighed by the benefits may require daily steroid therapy.

BW

182

Varicella

Chickenpox

In most persons specific antiviral therapy for varicella is not required. In certain risk groups (the immunosuppressed, neonates, and pregnant women with no prior history of varicella in the first trimester and within 5 days of delivery) therapy may be indicated. Consideration should also be given to passive immunization. Varicella pneumonia in the healthy adult should also be treated with acyclovir.

Initial Therapy

1. Not in a risk group: Tepid baths, oral antihistamines for pruritus, topical calamine lotion, and oral acetaminophen for fever.
2. Risk groups: Intravenous acyclovir 10 mg/kg t.i.d. for 7–10 days. In pregnant women, a dose of 7.5 mg/kg t.i.d. has been recommended.

3. All high-risk individuals with certain types of exposures should receive varicella-zoster immune globulin (VZIG) within the first 96 hours after exposure. If VZIG cannot be obtained within this time frame intravenous gamma globulin may be substituted.

Alternative Therapy

Risk groups: Intravenous vidarabine 10 mg/kg/day for 5–10 days.

Pitfalls

1. Secondary staphylococcal infection of varicella is common, and may be easily overlooked.
2. Reye syndrome may follow varicella, especially in children in whom aspirin is used as an antipyretic.
3. To avoid postvaricella scarring treat pruritus and secondary infection aggressively.

TB

183

Viral Exanthems

Viral exanthems are usually asymptomatic, and therapy usually is not required.

Initial Therapy (for Patients with Vesicobullous Lesions and/or Pruritus)

1. Antihistamines (e.g., hydroxyzine 10–25 mg t.i.d. or chlorpheniramine 4–16 mg/day) can be used to alleviate pruritus. For pediatric cases, hydroxyzine syrup or diphenhydramine elixir (1–2 tsp) q.h.s. can be used.
2. Tepid baths, with added oillated colloidal oatmeal (Aveeno), are useful for both relief of pruritus and debridement of vesicobullous lesions.
3. An antipruritic lotion containing menthol, camphor, and/or phenol (e.g., Sarna, Prax) can provide symptomatic relief.
4. See Chapter 87 for therapy of herpes simplex infections.

Pitfalls

1. Consider a drug eruption in the differential diagnosis in patients previously receiving drugs.
2. Antihistamines cause drowsiness, particularly during the first few days of therapy. Care must be taken in operating motor vehicles. Alcohol consumption can aggravate the drowsiness.
3. Arthritis and meningitis are rare complications of viral illnesses, although they occur with greater frequency in affected adults than children.
4. Viral exanthems can induce an aplastic crisis in patients with sickle cell anemia.

PE

184

Vitiligo

Vitiligo, a disorder of depigmentation, can be distinguished from disorders of hypopigmentation by its porcelain-white appearance (accentuated under Wood's light), its predilection for axial, acral, and periorificial areas, and the absence of any other skin changes. The course and extent of vitiligo are variable and unpredictable.

Initial Therapy

1. If patches cover only a small area, cosmetic masks (e.g., Dermablend or Covermark by Lydia O'Leary), available in most large department stores, should be employed.
2. A sunscreen with a SPF of 15 or greater should be employed to prevent both sunburn and skin cancer.
3. A minority of patients respond to topical therapy with a superpotent steroid cream, such as clobetasole diproprionate (Temovate). Facial lesions generally respond better (more than 90%) than lesions elsewhere (approximately 40%). For lesions on the eyelid, the ointment vehicle is preferred to minimize introduction of medication into the eyes. Once a response occurs (i.e., within 4–6 weeks) stop therapy, because repigmentation often continues to proceed. If only partial repigmentation occurs,

then a second and even a third course may be administered following a 4-month period of treatment.

Alternative Therapy

1. A medium-potency topical steroid may be helpful for limited numbers of lesions in a minority of patients (use low-potency steroids for intertriginous lesions).
2. Topical or systemic PUVA may be indicated to repigment patients with particularly disfiguring lesions. Refer patients to a physician with specific expertise with this therapy. Recently, phenylalamine has been substituted for psoralens with promising results and less phototoxicity (see *Archives of Dermatologic Research* 277:126–130, 1985).
3. In blacks with extensive, disfiguring vitiligo, total depigmentation with topical monobenzylether of hydroquinone can be considered. Again, this form of therapy should be administered by experts in the therapy of pigmentary abnormalities.
4. For stable vitiligo, unresponsive to topical steroids and/or photochemotherapy, autologous minigrafting may be successful (see *Archives of Dermatology 124:1649–1655, 1988).*

Subsequent Therapy/Work-up

A work-up beyond a careful review of symptoms is not indicated in asymptomatic patients. However, vitiligo is infrequently associated with mucocutaneous candidiasis, melanoma, and other autoimmune disorders (e.g., thyroiditis, diabetes, Addison's disease, and pernicious anemia). Obtain appropriate laboratory studies in patients with positive histories or examinations.

Pitfalls

1. If topical steroid therapy is undertaken, patients must be monitored for the development of cutaneous atrophy; and in any case, discontinue therapy after 4–6 weeks if no response is observed. Do not treat lesions in intertriginous areas, face, or genitalia, and do not administer this form of therapy to young children.
2. The risk of cataracts and sunburn in patients treated with PUVA is discussed in Chapter 147.
3. Monobenzylether of hydroquinone commonly causes an acute contact dermatitis.

PE

185

Warts

Verrucae

Human papillomavirus (HPV)-induced lesions (warts) are a common but vexing problem, as no ideal therapy exists. There are four basic types of warts: flat warts (verruca plana), common warts (verruca vulgaris), plantar warts, and genital warts (condyloma acuminata). The therapy of each wart type is discussed separately. Warts in the immunosuppressed are common, therapeutically difficult, and potentially oncogenic, and therefore are discussed separately. Epidermodysplasia verruciformis (EDV) appears to represent an unusual type of HPV-specific immunodeficiency. Squamous cell carcinoma of the skin occurs commonly from the warts in EDV in sun-exposed areas.

FLAT WARTS

Flat warts almost universally involute spontaneously over several months to years, with no sequelae. Therapy should be bland and nonscarring, as this is the expected result from spontaneous involution.

Initial Therapy

1. Retinoic acid 0.1% cream or 0.25% gel applied b.i.d. for 4–6 weeks to induce mild to moderate irritation will clear about 50% of patients.
2. Shaving over warts in the beard area or on the legs with a razor blade tends to spread the lesions. Males with warts in the beard, and women with warts on the legs, should not shave until the lesions are cleared. Electric shavers may reduce this spread.

Subsequent Therapy

1. For patients with a few lesions, light cryotherapy is quite effective, and may be used in conjunction with retinoic acid therapy.

2. Cantharidin (Cantharone, Verrusol) may be applied for 2–4 hours, without occlusion, then washed of with soap and water. Irritation and crusting of the warts is anticipated. Cantharidin is not to be used around the eyes.

Alternative Therapy

1. 5-Fluorouracil (5-FU) 5% cream may be applied to the affected area b.i.d. A brisk irritant reaction occurs at about 1 week, and warts resolve over 2–4 weeks. This therapy is highly effective, but is not recommended for children or pregnant women.
2. Formaldehyde 10%–20% in petrolatum may be applied b.i.d. Irritation is expected. This therapy is reserved for refractory cases, as allergic contact dermatitis may be induced. Formaldehyde is so ubiquitous that sensitivity to it may present a significant problem to the patient.

Pitfalls

1. In general, electrosurgery should be avoided for flat warts, as scarring occurs except when performed by the most expert hands.
2. Flat warts may be quite subtle and may be confused with inflammatory dermatoses. The application of topical steroids may potentially encourage spread of the warts, especially in atopics.

COMMON WARTS

Common (especially periungual) warts, are a challenge for even the most patient therapist. Although these warts will in general resolve spontaneously, the time course may be quite prolonged. Initial therapy should be as nontraumatic as possible, as all forms of treatment are associated with only about a 60%–70% success rate. Repeated applications of the same therapy may enhance the success rate. A positive attitude toward outcome on the part of the physician is very helpful. In children, this may be extended to suggestion therapy such as "buying" warts or taping warts with "special wart tape."

Initial Therapy

Cryotherapy with liquid nitrogen is effective, well tolerated (usually without anesthesia) and nonscarring if performed correctly. The iceball should extend 1–2 mm beyond the lesion, and thaw time should be between 30 and 45 seconds. Once thawed, the wart is frozen a second time in the same manner. Pain is moderate for about 5 minutes, and less severe for several hours. Analgesia with acetaminophen, aspirin, or a NSAID 30 minutes before the procedure improves patient tolerance. A blister, which may be hemorrhagic, should appear at 12–24 hours; its roof should be left intact as a dressing, but fluid may be drained if painful or if palmar/plantar pressure extends the blister. The patient should be seen at about 2–3 weeks or when the blister roof falls off. Earlier retreatment is more effective but also more uncomfortable. Initially, treatment is attempted at 2–3 weeks, but if this fails, retreat weekly. Remove all dead tissue before retreating.

Alternative Therapy

Keratolytics are painless and effective. Most contain salicylic acid and lactic acid (e.g., Duofilm 16.7% of each). Soak warts in warm water for 5 minutes, then dry the surface and apply the medication. Apply a Band-Aid for 24 hours as soon as the liquid dries. Repeat q.d. up to 6 weeks or until resolution. The response rate correlates with compliance, but averages about 50% for a single wart. This therapy may be combined with cryotherapy to treat any warts remaining after freezing.

Subsequent Therapy

1. Curettage of refractory acral lesions with or without shave biopsy of a portion for histopathologic evaluation may be useful. Local anesthesia (lidocaine) is required. Bleeding may be controlled with 20% aluminum chloride or very light electrodesiccation. *(Do not use local anesthetics containing epinephrine on acral lesions of the fingers or toes.)*
2. Cantharidin (Cantharone, Verrusol) is a blistering agent that may be painlessly applied by the physician in the office. It is good treatment for children unable to tolerate cryotherapy. Lesions are painted with the solution and covered with occlusive tape (Blenderm) when the solution has dried. The tape is then removed and the cantharidin washed off in 24 hours for acral nonperiungual, nonpalmar lesions, and in 48 hours for palmar and periungual lesions. Remove the dressing and wash off the medication

immediately if burning occurs prior to this time. A blister forms, and its roof dries and desquamates. Repeat biweekly or weekly for refractory lesions.

Therapy for Refractory Lesions

For the most difficult, unresponsive warts, referral to a specialist may be needed. Therapeutic options in this unusual group of patients include:

1. Bleomycin sulfate 0.1% (1 mg/cc) in normal saline may be injected into the wart(s). Usually less than 0.2 cc per lesion (until the lesion blanches) is required. Treatment may be repeated in 3 weeks for a total of 2–3 treatments. A success rate of 75%–95% is expected for acral common warts. The solution is very expensive, but stable for 60 days in the refrigerator (4°C) if kept sterile.
2. Immunotherapy with dinitrochlorobenzene after sensitization or by application of another known allergen to the wart (e.g., *Rhus* extract) may lead to wart resolution. An allergic dermatitis is anticipated over the wart; applications are repeated at the frequency and concentration required to maintain the dermatitis or until the wart(s) resolve. If the reaction wanes, cimetidine 200 mg q.i.d. may be added.
3. Carbon dioxide laser ablation of all of the wart, including a 1–2-mm rim of normal skin, gives a high cure rate. The high cost may be a drawback.
4. In exceptional cases oral retinoids may be useful.

Pitfalls

1. Recurrence is common, and does not mandate changing the therapeutic regimen.
2. Cryotherapy may lead to scarring and hypopigmentation, particularly in blacks and orientals, usually resolving over time.
3. Patients with Raynaud's, cryoglobulinemia, and severe peripheral vascular diseases should not have cryotherapy.
4. Keratolytics, if not applied carefully and allowed to dry thoroughly before bandaging, may erode adjacent skin.
5. In rare cases, a ring of warts (doughnut wart) will appear peripheral to the resolved wart.
6. Curettage, and especially electrodesiccation and CO_2 laser ablation, may

cause more scarring than cryotherapy. Hypopigmentation also may occur, especially in pigmented individuals.

7. Bleomycin injections are often painful and may cause a florid inflammatory response, blackening of the wart, erosion, or ulceration. Acral lesions should be treated with care owing to the possibility of persistent digital vasospasm or Raynaud's phenomenon.

8. The induction of an allergic contact dermatitis on the warts may be followed by a dyshidrosiform hand dermatitis or a generalized eruption. Allergen-treated sites should be occluded to prevent spread to distant sites.

9. Electrosurgery and the CO_2 laser generate a smokey plume that may contain infectious viral particles. The operator may be at risk of infection unless a well-fitted, filtered mask is worn and the smoke rapidly evacuated.

10. For side effects of oral retinoids, see Appendix 6.

PLANTAR WARTS

Plantar warts are difficult to treat. Curing 50% of plantar warts by any method is considered a good result. Overaggressive treatment should be avoided, as a plantar scar may be permanently painful.

Initial Therapy

Salicylic acid 40% plasters (e.g., Mediplast) applied q.d. under an occlusive dressing (adhesive tape) after soaking the warts in warm water for 10–15 minutes and scraping off dead tissue leads to gradual resolution of the lesion. Treatment is continued until the normal skin lines return in the wart-affected areas. A new salicylic acid 27% gel (Duoplast), or standard keratolytics (Duofilm), may be applied as alternatives. Apply after soaking the warts 5–10 minutes, then cover with an adhesive; repeat q.d. until resolution.

Alternative Therapy

1. Cryotherapy, repeated at 1–3-week intervals to generate a blister (as noted above), is safe and effective; several treatments are usually required. The blister roof is removed before retreating.

2. For extensive mosaic warts, soak in formalin 4% solution 15 minutes q.d. or apply formalin 10%–20% ointment q.d.

3. Cantharidin (Cantharone, Verrusol) may be applied for 24–48 hours to induce blister formation beneath and around the wart. Treatment is repeated at 1–3-week intervals, after debridement of the blistered tissue.

Subsequent Therapy

Blunt dissection, or enucleation with a curette can be used to remove the wart after local or regional anesthesia. Aluminum chloride is used for hemostasis. If done correctly, this is nonscarring and effective.

Therapy for Refractory Lesions

Bleomycin injections, or CO_2 laser therapy as described above for refractory common warts, may also be used on plantar warts. Cure rates are in the 50%–75% range.

Pitfalls

1. Overaggressive therapy of plantar warts may lead to persistent painful scars on the sole.
2. Salicylic acid plasters will also dissolve normal stratum corneum, so the plasters should be applied only to the wart and a very thin rim of normal skin to avoid excess irritation.
3. Contact allergy to formaldehyde appearing as a pruritic rash may develop during formalin treatment.
4. For complications of bleomycin therapy and CO_2 laser treatment, see Common Warts above.

GENITAL WARTS

Comments

1. Genital warts should be considered a STD. Evaluation for other STDs and simultaneous evaluation, with treatment of infected sexual contacts, is required.
2. In women, and less commonly in men, genital warts are potentially oncogenic. For *females*, a complete pelvic examination with a 5–10-minute soaking of the cervix and vagina with 3%–5% acetic acid (household white vinegar), a colposcopy, and a Pap smear are recommended. For this

reason, referral of these patients to a gynecologist for management is preferred. For *males,* 3%–5% acetic acid soaks of the genitals followed by examination with magnification under good light is suggested. Genital warts appear whiter than normal skin (mucosa), hence *acetowhite.* Not all acetowhite lesions are warts. A biopsy of atypical lesions is suggested in those patients without a prior history of genital warts, or if typical genital warts are not present elsewhere. This is especially true for flat (macular) lesions.

3. For perianal warts, proctoscopy concurrent with the treatment of external warts is essential to detect associated internal warts.

4. Genital warts in children (especially those in whom the warts appear after 6 months of age) require an evaluation for sexual abuse. Evidence of sexual child abuse is found in up to 50% of cases.

5. Atypical, flat, and pigmented condylomata may suggest the diagnosis of Bowenoid papulosis. A biopsy should be performed. This is often associated with HPV 16, and histologically may show features of squamous cell carcinoma in situ. Total eradication of these lesions should be attempted. They are treated in the same manner as genital warts. 5-Fluorouracil (5-FU) and electrosurgery have been most effective in our patients.

6. Eradication of extensive genital warts in males and females is extremely difficult. Spontaneous resolution is rare, and sexual transmission is common. Because genital HPV infection is clearly linked to genital squamous cell carcinoma, total eradication should be attempted.

Initial Therapy

Only the treatment of external genital and perianal condylomata are discussed here.

1. Treat external genital and perianal condyloma acuminata with podophyllin 25% in tincture of benzoin. Avoiding normal skin, use cotton-tip applicators to apply small amounts to the warts only; blot off any podophyllin that runs onto noninfected skin with a fresh, dry applicator. The patient washes off the podophyllin in 4–8 hours, or when burning occurs. This is repeated weekly until the lesions are totally resolved (usually after 6–10 treatments). Podophyllin works best in moist, occluded areas. It should not be used during pregnancy, in infants, or on the vagina or cervix.

2. Cryotherapy is more often effective than podophyllin but also more painful. In dry areas, such as the penile shaft, it is an appropriate initial therapy. It may also be used on other condylomata that have not responded to podophyllin or trichloroacetic acid. Totally freeze each wart, allowing the iceball to extend 2 mm beyond the wart; freeze a second time after the wart is thawed. Repeat treatments at 1–2-week intervals.

Alternative Therapy

Trichloroacetic acid (TCA) 50%–75% may be applied cautiously to warts as for podophyllin, using the wooden end of the applicator; avoid contact with visibly uninfected surfaces. Cure rates are similar to podophyllin.

Subsequent Therapy

For condylomata not responding to repeated podophyllin/TCA and cryotherapy. (There is no absolute definition for "nonresponders"; failure after 10 weekly treatments suggests the use of alternative treatments.)

1. Electrosurgery, after local anesthesia with lidocaine 1% with epinephrine, is very effective for refractory warts. Penile shaft and perianal warts respond especially well. *(Do not use local anesthetics containing epinephrine on acral lesions of the penis.)* Each wart is totally ablated with electrodesiccation. Healing is usually rapid. Due to the pain of local anesthetic injection, only a limited number of warts can be treated at each visit. Sodium bicarbonate buffering of the lidocaine (1 part sodium bicarbonate 8.4% to 10 parts lidocaine 1% or 2%, with or without epinephrine) reduces the discomfort of the injection. Lidocaine buffered in this fashion is unstable, and must be remade daily.

2. Topical 5% 5-Fluorouracil (5-FU) has efficacy in several settings in managing condylomata.
   a. Distal urethral meatus warts are treated by injecting a small volume (0.5–3 cc) of 5% cream via syringe (minus needle) into the urethra b.i.d. or t.i.d. for 2–3 weeks. Dysuria is common, but can usually be tolerated by the patient; if pain is severe, urinating with the penis in warm water (bath, bowl) may help.
   b. Attempts have been made to treat other external genital condylomata with 5-FU. Optimal dose and regimen have not been determined. The 5% cream is applied b.i.d. for 2–3 weeks. Excessive irritation of unaffected skin, especially of the scrotum, has occurred and the warts have often not responded.
   c. Bowenoid papulosis often responds quite well to topical 5-FU b.i.d. for 3–4 weeks.
   d. Infection by HPV of apparently normal skin is common, especially in patients with extensive condylomata. Therefore, once these patients appear clinically cleared, topical 5-FU cream may be applied once or twice weekly in an attempt to prevent relapse. The efficacy of, and optimal regimen for, this treatment has not yet been established.

3. Intralesional α interferon has been approved to treat limited numbers of condylomata. In a published study the cure rate for *individual* warts was 73%, and total wart resolution occurred in 62% of patients, compared to placebo-treated cure rates of 36% and 21%, respectively. Each wart is injected directly and at its margins with 0.05 to 0.1 cc/25 mm^2. A total of 0.5 cc per visit is allowed. Injections are repeated biweekly for 8 weeks until resolution of the treated warts. Therapy produces significant side effects (fever, flu-like illness, malaise) in a large number of patients. Due to the high cost and the limited numbers of warts that can be treated, this therapy currently appears to have limited usefulness.

Refractory and Extensive Warts

Extensive condylomata are very difficult to eradicate by any method. These patients are best referred to persons experienced in their treatment.

1. Carbon dioxide (CO_2) laser ablation is the most effective surgical method available. If extensive, however, general or spinal anesthesia may be required. Recovery requires at least 1 week.
2. Intramuscular (systemic) interferon has been effective, but side effects are common. This is still considered experimental therapy in the United States.

Pitfalls

1. Podophyllin if not removed can cause severe cutaneous and mucosal erosions. If treating under the foreskin, treat only 50% of the circumference at a time. Too aggressive treatment can lead to phimosis, which may require a dorsal slit. Podophyllin should not be used in pregnancy, on infants, in the vagina, or on the cervix.
2. Trichloroacetic acid may cause severe genital erosions if not used cautiously. Local severe reactions may mimic microbial cellulitis.
3. Blisters may occur following cryotherapy, and overaggressive treatment may lead to scarring.
4. Electrosurgery usually leaves small scars, which may be dyspigmented.
5. 5-FU regularly causes irritant dermatitis if applied too frequently or to thin-skinned areas (e.g., scrotum).
6. Interferon injections for intralesional or systemic therapy cause flu-like symptoms and fevers in the majority of patients.
7. Potentially infectious viral particles are present in both electrosurgical and laser smoke plumes. Filtered masks should be used, in addition to a smoke evacuation system.

8. Not all verrucous or acetowhite lesions on the genitals are warts. Consider also pearly penile papules, condylomata lata (secondary syphilis), and molluscum contagiosum. If in doubt, biopsy the lesions or seek additional consultations.

WARTS IN THE IMMUNOSUPPRESSED/ EPIDERMODYSPLASIA VERRUCIFORMIS

All of the modalities outlined above *except interferon* appear to be useful, but of reduced efficacy, in immunosuppressed patients (interferon does not appear to work in this context). Oral retinoids may also be used in epidermodysplasia verruciformis therapy, but high doses are required, and relapse universally occurs when these agents are discontinued. Since immunosuppressed patients often cannot be cured of their warts, special care must be paid to the association of warts and squamous cell carcinoma. The progression of warts to cancer appears to be accelerated. Sun exposure is an important cofactor in nongenital cutaneous lesions.

1. For genital warts in women, a regular Pap smear and colposcopy are suggested. Men with genital warts should be followed closely as well. Any suspicious or large lesion must be biopsied.
2. Sun protection must include total covering of the arms, legs, and head with clothing. In addition, a broad-spectrum, high-SPF sunscreen must be applied q.d. to the face, neck, ears, and arms, as some UV light does go through loosely knit clothing. Any suspicious, nonhealing, and nonresolving lesion should be biopsied.

TB

186

Xanthomas

Multiple xanthomas almost always indicate an inherited or acquired hyperlipidemic state. However, xanthomas rarely occur in normolipenic individuals, and xanthelasma is common in normolipenic individuals. In such cases hypolipidemic therapy is not helpful. Treatment of the primary hyperlipidemias should be undertaken with the assistance of an endocrine-metabolism consultant.

Initial Therapy

1. A diagnostic laboratory work-up is mandatory, and in some cases is urgent, as in eruptive xanthomas associated with diabetic ketoacidosis. A minimal lipid profile includes fasting serum cholesterol, triglycerides, LDL, HDL, and VLDL. Ultracentrifugation techniques have replaced electrophoresis for the quantitation of serum lipoproteins. Other studies that should be obtained are fasting and postprandial blood glucose levels, thyroid function studies, BUN and creatinine, LFTs, uric acid, and a routine urinalysis.
2. In primary lipidemias, dietary therapy is the mainstay of therapy.
   a. Reduction of weight toward normal is essential.
   b. Reduction in intake of total calories, particularly in the form of carbohydrates and alcohol, is critical for reduction of hypertriglyceridemia.
   c. Reduction in dietary cholesterol to less than 300 mg/day is indicated for patients with hypercholesterolemia.
3. Drug therapy should be implemented only when dietary measures do not suffice, and only in conjunction with appropriate dietary restriction.
   a. For hypertriglyceridemia (type III, IV, or V hyperlipoproteinemias), both clofibrate (Atromid S) 500 mg q.i.d. and gemfibrozil (Lopid) 900–1500 mg/day in a b.i.d. dosage, taken 30 minutes before the morning and evening meal, are effective. Gemfibrozil is preferred when hypertriglyceridemia is accompanied by significant hypercholesterolemia.
   b. For hypercholesterolemia, several different classes of agents are available, but the inhibitor of HMGCoA reductase, lovastatin (Mevaacor), is the most effective and best-tolerated agent. Begin with lovastatin 20 mg/day, and increase to 80 mg/day p.r.n.

Ancillary Therapy

1. In addition to dietary restrictions and weight reduction, patients with hyperlipidemia should be instructed to stop smoking.
2. Adequate physical exercise also helps lower blood lipid levels.
3. Persistent individual xanthomas, such as in normolipemic xanthelasma, can be chemically cauterized with trichloracetic acid 35%, applied to the xanthoma only, with a cotton-tipped applicator. Therapy can be repeated on a biweekly basis until lesions are flat.

Alternative (or Combination) Therapy

1. Nicotinic acid, beginning with 500 mg t.i.d., increasing by one pill each day to a total of 3–4.5 g/day, is a useful alternative to lovastatin for hypercholesterolemia, and will reduce triglycerides somewhat, as well. Nicotinic acid should be taken at end of meals and without alcohol or hot foods to reduce flushing (see Pitfalls).
2. Cholestyramine (Questran) powder, 1 4-g scoopful with breakfast and 2 scoops with dinner, increasing to 3 scoops b.i.d., is an effective alternative for patients unable to tolerate lovastatin or nicotinic acid.

Pitfalls

1. Patients with hypertriglyceridemia in excess of 1,000 mg% are at risk for acute pancreatitis. Hence, therapy should be implemented quickly.
2. Xanthomas can be the presenting feature of several underlying systemic diseases, ranging from nephrotic syndrome to primary biliary cirrhosis. If the search for these causes is productive, therapy of the underlying problem then should eliminate the xanthomas.
3. Because both gemfibrozil and clofibrate are excreted via the kidneys, dosages need to be adjusted in patients with renal disease.
4. Because both gemfibrozil and clofibrate interfere with coagulation in patients on oral anticoagulants, prothrombin times must be checked frequently, and the anticoagulant dose adjusted accordingly.
5. A statistically significant increase in cholecystitis, pancreatitis, and malignancy has been reported in patients on long-term therapy with clofibrate or gemfibrozil.
6. Cholestyramine can produce both upper and lower GI side effects (bloating and constipation); antacids and/or laxatives may be required.
7. The flushing associated with nicotinic acid use often can be prevented by coadministration of aspirin, 1–6 tablets/day.
8. Lovastatin rarely can cause abnormal LFTs and a myositis-like syndrome. Because this class of agents still is relatively new, other long-term effects could still appear.

PE

187

Xerosis

Xerosis can reflect an inherited tendency toward dry skin (e.g., as a part of the atopic diathesis), or it can occur in normal individuals as a consequence of frequent bathing with excessively hot water and harsh soaps and/or after prolonged exposure to unusually low environmental humidities (as occurs with forced-air heating during winter months in cold climates). Finally, xerosis can occur as a consequence of asteatosis (e.g., with suppression of sebaceous gland function during isotretinoin (Accutane) therapy of acne). Whether xerosis occurs solely as a natural consequence of aging is not known, but it seems clear that normal aging is at least a predisposing factor.

Initial Therapy

1. Reduce the frequency of bathing, and reduce the temperature of the water. *Note:* The frequency of bathing is not as critical as reduction of the water temperature. However, overly compulsive bathers should be encouraged to bathe less frequently.
2. Use of mild soaps. Dove is the least expensive of the oilated soaps, which generally are at least as useful as glycerinated soaps.
3. For patients who take tub baths, an oilated solution such as Alpha-Keri, Domol, or colloidal oatmeal (Aveeno) can be added. *Note:* Older persons are particularly at risk of slipping in the tub, so patients should be warned and appropriate precautions should be taken (e.g., use a rubber bath mat).
4. *Immediately* after bathing, an emollient cream or ointment (e.g., aqua-aquaphor (Eucerin), petrolatum (Vaseline), or Nivea) should be applied to xerotic skin surfaces and rubbed in well while skin is still damp.

Subsequent Therapy

1. Recalcitrant xerosis with secondary pruritus can be the harbinger of systemic disease. If the above, intensive protocol does not bring relief in 2–3 weeks, a search for an underlying metabolic or neoplastic cause should be instituted.
2. Antihistamines may be helpful adjuncts to the management of itch, but should be used with caution in the elderly due to additive sedative effects of

multiple medications, and/or anticholinergic side effects, including urinary retention, precipitation of closed-angle glaucoma, and supraventricular tachycardias (all rare). Nevertheless, antihistamines should be given q.h.s. only, or in very low doses initially.

3. If several members of a household all have xerosis or other dry skin-related problems, a cool-air vaporizer in the bedroom or other living areas can be useful during winter months to counteract the low humidities of closed-air heating systems.

4. The symptoms of xerosis tend to vary in severity with the season, therefore, the intensity of management should take these seasonal variations into account.

Pitfalls

1. If left untreated, xerotic skin may become eczematous, resulting in erythema, increased pruritus, and occasionally, nummular dermatitis.

2. The recent onset of generalized xerosis, with or without pruritus, can reflect underlying metabolic or neoplastic disease (see above).

3. The potential pitfalls of antihistamine therapy, especially in the elderly, are discussed above.

PE

Appendix 1

Topical Steroids: Available Formulations and Their Costs[a]

Steroid	Cost	Range	Vehicle
Lowest potency[b]			
Dexamethasone 0.1%	7.88		Cream
Decadron Phosphate (Merck)			
Decarderm (Merck)	8.12		Gel
Hydrocortisone 1%	1.77	1.20–2.88	Cream
Average generic price	1.77	1.20–2.88	Ointment
			Lotion

(Continued)

Steroid	Cost	Range	Vehicle
Average name brand price	2.17	1.13–5.04	Cream
	n/a		Ointment
	1.65	0.50–5.27	Lotion
Cort-Dome (Miles)	7.62		Cream
Cortef Acetate (Upjohn)	10.00		Ointment
Penecort (Herbert)	1.85		Cream
Hydrocortisone 2.5%	2.71	1.91–3.41	Cream
Average generic price			
Average name brand price	3.48	3.41–4.07	Cream
Penecort (Herbert)	3.34		Cream
Synacort (Syntex)	3.52		Cream
Hytone (Dermik)	4.07		Ointment
Methylprednisolone acetate 0.25%	5.34		Ointment
Medrol (Upjohn)			
Methylprednisolone acetate 1%	10.60		Ointment
Medrol (Upjohn)			
Low potency[b]			
Alclometasone 0.05%	7.56		Cream, ointment
Aclovate (Glaxo)			
Clocortolone 0.1%	7.70		Cream
Clorderm (Herman)			
Desonide 0.05%	6.72		Cream
Desowen (Owen)			
Tridesilon (Miles)	7.61		Cream, ointment
Fluocinolone acetonide 0.01%	1.45	1.00–2.04	Cream
Average generic price			
Synalar (Syntex)	5.58		Cream
Fluandrenolide 0.025%	4.29		Cream, ointment
Cordran, Cordran SP (Dista)			
Triamcinolone acetonide 0.025%	1.09	0.80–1.78	Cream
Average generic price			Ointment
			Lotion
Average name brand price			Cream
Aristocort (Lederle)	4.48		Cream
Aristocort A (Lederle)	6.58		Cream
Kenalog (Squibb)	4.68		Cream, ointment
Intermediate potency[c]			
Betamethasone benzoate 0.025%	4.44		Lotion, gel, ointment
Benisone (Rydell)			
(60 g)	11.83		Cream
Uticort (Parke-Davis)	6.46		Gel, lotion
	17.16		Cream

(Continued)

Steroid	Cost	Range	Vehicle
Betamethasone valerate 0.1%	3.07	2.00 4.40	Cream
Average generic price	3.19	2.16–4.63	Ointment
	2.27	1.63–3.49	Lotion
Average brand-name price			Cream, ointment
			Lotion
Valisone (Schering)	8.70		Cream, ointment
	8.06		Lotion
Desoximetasone 0.05%	6.65		Cream
Topicort (Hoechst-Roussel)	7.50		Gel
Fluocinolone acetonide 0.025%	2.17	1.25–4.50	Cream, ointment
Average generic price			Cream
Average brand-name price			Ointment
Fluonid (Herbert)	8.94		Cream
			Ointment
Synalar (Syntex)	n/a		Cream/ointment
Fluandrenolide 0.05%	3.44	3.15–3.74	Lotion
Average generic price			
Cordran, Cordran SP (Dista)	7.74		Cream,ointment
			Lotion
Halcinonide 0.025%	7.36		Cream
Halog (Princeton)			
Mometasone furoate 0.1%	8.70		Cream, ointment
Elocon (Schering)			
Triamcinolone acetonide 0.1%	1.49	0.91–2.56	Cream, ointment
Average generic price	2.34	1.22–4.05	Lotion
Average brand-name price			Cream
			Ointment
Aristocort (Lederle)	5.66		Cream, ointment
Aristocort A (Lederle)	7.02		Cream, ointment
Kenalog (Squibb)	5.57		Cream, ointment
			Lotion
High Potency[d]			
Amcionide 0.1%	9.26		Cream, ointment
Cyclocort (Lederle)			
Betamethasone dipropionate 0.05%	4.95	3.40–6.60	Cream, ointment
Average generic price			
	2.67	2.15–3.26	Lotion
Alphatrex (Savage)	6.62		Cream, ointment
(60 ml)	15.50		Lotion
Diprosone (Schering)	11.04		Cream, ointment
(20 ml)	13.56		Lotion
Desoximetasone 0.25%	8.70		Cream, ointment
Topicort (Hoechst-Roussel)	n/a		Gel

(Continued)

Steroid	Cost	Range	Vehicle
Difluorasone diacetate 0.05%	8.41		Cream, ointment
Florone (Dermik)			
Maxifluor (Herbert) (30 mg)	9.45		Cream, ointment
Fluocinolone 0.2%	15.29		Cream
Synalar HP (Syntex) (12 g)			
Fluocinonide 0.05%	14.36		Cream, gel, ointment
Lidex, Lidex-E (Syntex) (30 g)			
Halcinonide 0.1%	15.70		Cream, ointment
Halog, Halog-E (Squibb) (30 g)	11.71		Solution
Triamcinolone acetonide 0.5%	3.41	2.37–5.19	Cream, ointment
Average generic price			
Average brand-name price			Cream
Aristocort A (Lederle) (15 g)	22.90		Cream
Aristocrat (Lederle) (15 g)	18.23		Cream, ointment
Kenalog (Squibb) (20 g)	22.29		Cream, ointment
Super potency[d]			
Betamethasone dipropionate 0.05%	12.91		Cream, ointment
Diprolene (Schering)			
Clobetasol propionate 0.05%	17.86		Cream, ointment
Temovate (Glaxo)			
Diflorasone diacetate 0.05%	14.26		Ointment
Psorcon (Dermik)			

[a] Based on manufacturers listing in *Drug Topics Red Book 1988.* Average wholesale price used when available. Cost to patient will be higher.

[b] Cost of 15g to the pharmacist.

[c] Cost of 15g (cream or ointment) or 15 ml (lotion) to the pharmacist.

[d] Cost of 30g (cream or ointment) to the pharmacist.

n/a, not available.

Appendix 2

Topical Antifungal Agents

(See table on next page.)

Active Ingredient	Proprietary Name	Preparation	How Supplied
Polyenes			
Amphotericin B	Fungizone	3% Cream	20 g
		3% Lotion	30 ml
		3% Ointment	20 g
Nystatin	Candex	Powder (100,000 U/g)	0.5 oz.
		Suspension (100,000 U/ml)	5 ml, 60 ml, 473 ml
		Tablets (500,000 U)	100
	Mycostatin	Cream (100,000 U/g)	15 g, 30 g
	Nystex	Ointment (100,000 U/g)	15 g, 30 g
Imidazoles			
Clotrimazole	Lotrimin	1% Cream	15 g, 30 g
			45 g, 90 g
	Mycelex	1% Lotion	30 ml
		1% Solution	10 ml, 30 ml
		Tablets (100 mg)	6 or 7/package
Econazole	Spectazol	1% Cream	15 g, 30 g, 85 g
Miconazole	Micatin	2% Cream	15 g, 1 oz., 3 oz.
	Monistat	2% Lotion	30 ml, 60 ml
		2% Powder	1.5 oz.
		Suppository (100 mg)	3 or 7/package
Miscellaneous			
Chlordantoin	Sporostacin		
Ciclopirox olamine	Loprox	1% Cream	15 g, 30 g
Haloprogin	Halotex	1% Cream	15 g, 30 g
		1% Solution	10 ml, 30 ml
Iodochlorhydroxyquin	Vioform	3% Ointment	1 oz.
		3% Cream	1 oz.

(From Bodey GP: Topical and systemic antifungal agents. Med Clin North Am 72(3):637, 1988, with permission.)

Appendix 3

Pitfalls of Topical Corticosteroid Therapy

Topical steroid side effects are both local (cutaneous) and systemic. The greater the potency of the steroid and the greater the amount applied, the greater is the likelihood of side effects. The use of occlusion also makes side effects more likely.

1. Vasoconstriction with local pallor may occur within hours of application of topical steroids, but reverses in 48 hours or sooner when application is discontinued.
2. Hypopigmentation may occur in dark-skinned patients, but is reversible with discontinuation or reduction of strength.
3. Acne may be produced in a susceptible individual by steroid application to susceptible sites (face, upper trunk). Acne rosaccea may be induced or exacerbated by topical steroids at medium potency or stronger. Perioral dermatitis is a form of steroid induced rosacea around the mouth or eyes.
4. Atrophy and striae occur with the chronic use of medium-potency or stronger steroids in occluded areas (groin, axilla, neck) or when using mechanical occlusion (plastic wrap). Superpotent steroids may induce these changes on almost all cutaneous surfaces if used chronically.
5. Telangiectasis may result from chronic steroid use on the face, especially in persons with rosacea.
6. Purpura may occur in atrophic skin (e.g., from chronic sun damage in the elderly).
7. Allergic contact dermatitis to steroid preparations may rarely occur, either from the vehicle or from the active agent itself.
8. Tinea and candida may be masked or enhanced by topical steroid application. This may particularly be a problem in cases of tinea cruris, where combined steroid-antiyeast preparations (e.g., Mycolog) or steroid-antifungal preparations (e.g., Lotrisone) tend to be used inappropriately.
9. Glaucoma and cataracts may occur with topical applications on or around the eyelids. It is best to avoid using all topical steroids between the supra- and infraorbital rims, and between the medial and lateral canthi. If steroids must be used on the eyelid, only hydrocortisone 1% or less is recommended.
10. Suppression of the pituitary-adrenal axis may occur with sufficient topical steroid application, especially if applied under occlusion or to exten-

sively inflamed skin. Enough steroid may be absorbed to produce Cushing's syndrome.

Appendix 4

Pitfalls of Intralesional Corticosteroid Therapy

1. Local atrophy is the most common side effect of intralesional steroid therapy. Too much steroid by volume or concentration usually causes this complication. Injection in the fat regularly leads to fat atrophy, which may persist for years. Injections that were too superficial in the dermis may lead to visible steroid deposits and persistent atrophy.
2. Atrophy along draining lymphatics may occur, especially when acral injections are given.
3. Hypopigmentation occurs most commonly in dark-skinned individuals, and resolves, slowly.
4. Rarely, intralesional injections on the head, especially around the eyes, may cause temporary or permanent blindness (amaurosis fugax) owing to embolization of steroid particles in the retinal vessels.

Appendix 5

Pitfalls of Systemic Steroids

FREQUENT COMPLICATIONS

1. Sodium and fluid retention, potassium loss, hypertension, and congestive heart failure. To avoid these complications, monitor blood pressure,

weight, and serum potassium in patients receiving long-term steroid therapy.
2. Peptic ulcer with possible hemorrhage or perforation. Patients with a history of peptic ulcer disease should regularly use antacids. Consider therapy with an H_2 antagonist.
3. Psychic derangements. Patients treated acutely with high-dose systemic steroids should be warned about this common complication of therapy.
4. Carbohydrate intolerance. Prior to high-dose therapy, patients should be questioned with regard to a personal or family history of diabetes. After 2 weeks of steroid therapy and when the steroid dose is stabilized in patients on long-term therapy, obtain a fasting blood glucose level. Particular care should be taken in patients with a family history of diabetes.

OTHER COMPLICATIONS

1. Steroid myopathy and loss of muscle mass.
2. Osteoporosis and vertebral compression fractures; aseptic necrosis of the femoral heads, and pathologic fracture of long bone.
3. Pancreatitis.
4. Ulcerative esophagitis.
5. Fragile skin, petechiae and ecchymoses, impaired wound healing, facial telangiectasia.
6. Increased intracranial pressure with papilledema, headache.
7. Menstrual irregularities.
8. Cushingoid state.
9. Growth impairment.
10. Adrenocortical suppression.
11. Posterior subcapsular cataracts.
12. Glaucoma.
13. Exophthalmus.
14. Opportunistic infection associated with chronic immunosuppression.

Appendix 6

Pitfalls of Systemic Retinoid Therapy

1. Almost all patients experience mild mucocutaneous side effects.
2. More serious potential problems include:
   a. Ocular disorders (cataracts, night blindness).
   b. Hepatic disorders (chemical hepatitis).
   c. Teratogenicity (these drugs are absolutely contraindicated for women of child-bearing potential who are not on an effective form of birth control).
   d. Most importantly, musculoskeletal disorders (diffuse idiopathic skeletal hyperostosis [DISH syndrome], calcification of ligaments and tendons, or acceleration of pre-existing bone or joint disease). Musculoskeletal toxicity occurs in 20%–40% of patients undergoing more than 6 months of therapy with doses greater than 1 mg/kg/day of either retinoid, and can progress even after discontinuation of drug.
3. Premature closure of the epiphyses can occur in young children treated with retinoids.
4. Hypertriglyceridemia and hypercholesterolemia occur in a substantial number of patients, therefore, fasting serum lipids must be evaluated regularly during systemic retinoid therapy. Minor increases in serum lipids do not necessarily dictate cessation of therapy; weight reduction and cessation of smoking and/or alcohol consumption may suffice to normalize serum lipids, even with ongoing therapy.

Appendix 7

Pitfalls of Chemotherapeutic Agents Used in Dermatologic Therapy

METHOTREXATE

1. Frequent complications are ulcerative stomatitis, leukopenia, nausea, and abdominal distress
2. Less frequent complications include:
   a. Pruritus and photosensitivity.
   b. Gingivitis, pharyngitis, vomiting, diarrhea, hematemesis, melena, and GI ulceration.
   c. Renal failure.
   d. Transient oligospermia.
   e. Menstrual dysfunction, infertility, abortion, and fetal defects.
   f. Interstitial pneumonitis.
   g. Headaches, drowsiness, and blurred vision.

AZATHIOPRINE (IMURAN)

1. Frequent complications include:
   a. Reversible, dose-dependent leukopenia and thrombocytopenia.
   b. Nausea and vomiting, reduced by administration in divided dosage or after meals.
2. Less frequent complications include:
   a. Hepatotoxicity, detected by elevation of serum alkaline phosphatase and transaminases.
   b. Alopecia.
   c. Fever and arthralgias.
   d. Diarrhea.
   e. Steatorrhea.
   f. Fetal malformations.

CYCLOPHOSPHAMIDE (CYTOXAN)

1. Development of malignancies, including lymphoproliferative disorders and urinary bladder malignancies in individuals who previously had hemorrhagic cystitis.

2. Fetal abnormalities.
3. Sterility in both sexes.
4. Nausea and vomiting.
5. Alopecia and pigmentary alterations.
6. Leukopenia and thrombocytopenia.
7. Hemorrhagic cystitis. To avoid this complication, increased fluid intake should be during the day so that the cyclophosphamide does not remain in the bladder overnight or for prolonged periods of time.
8. Interstitial pulmonary fibrosis.

Appendix 8

Abbreviations Used in the Text

AIDS	Acquired immunodeficiency syndrome
ANA	Antinuclear antibody
ARC	AIDS-related complex
b.i.d.	Two times daily
BUN	Blood urea nitrogen
CBC	Complete blood count
CDC	Centers for Disease Control
CNS	Central nervous system
CSF	Cerebral spinal fluid
CT	Computed tomography
ECG	Electrocardiogram
ESR	Erythrocyte sedimentation rate
FDA	Food & Drug Administration
GI	Gastrointestinal
G6PD	Glucose-6-phosphate dehydrogenase
GU	Genitourinary
HDL	High-density lipoprotein
HIV	Human immunodeficiency virus
KOH	Potassium hydroxide
LDL	Low-density lipoprotein
LFT	Liver function test

MRI	Magnetic resonance imaging
NSAID	Nonsteroidal anti-inflammatory drug
OCP	Oral contraceptive pill
PDR	Physician's Desk Reference
p.o.	Orally
p.r.n.	As needed
PUVA	Psoralens plus ultraviolet A
q.a.m.	Every morning
q.d.	Daily
q.h.s.	At bedtime
q.i.d.	Four times daily
q.o.d.	Every other day
q.o.h.s.	Every other night at bedtime
STD	Sexually transmitted disease
TFT	Thyroid function test
t.i.d	Three times daily
tsp	Teaspoon
VLDL	Very low-density lipoprotein
WBC	White blood cell count

Index

Page numbers followed by *t* indicate tables.